Marketing Chiropractic to Medical Practices

Christina L. Acampora, DC

Member
American Chiropractic Association
Foundation for Chiropractic Education and Research

Founder
Aligned Methods
Chicago, Illinois

JONES AND BARTLETT PUBLISHERS
Sudbury, Massachusetts
BOSTON   TORONTO   LONDON   SINGAPORE

World Headquarters

Jones and Bartlett Publishers
40 Tall Pine Drive
Sudbury, MA 01776
978-443-5000
info@jbpub.com
www.jbpub.com

Jones and Bartlett Publishers
Canada
6339 Ormindale Way
Mississauga, Ontario L5V 1J2
CANADA

Jones and Bartlett Publishers
International
Barb House, Barb Mews
London W6 7PA
UK

Jones and Bartlett's books and products are available through most bookstores and online book-sellers. To contact Jones and Bartlett Publishers directly, call 800-832-0034, fax 978-443-8000, or visit our website www.jbpub.com.

Substantial discounts on bulk quantities of Jones and Bartlett's publications are available to corporations, professional associations, and other qualified organizations. For details and specific discount information, contact the special sales department at Jones and Bartlett via the above contact information or send an email to specialsales@jbpub.com.

This publication is designed to provide accurate and authoritative information in regard to the subject matter covered. It is sold with the understanding that the publisher is not engaged in rendering legal, accounting, or other professional service. If legal advice or other expert assistance is required, the service of a competent professional person should be sought.

Library of Congress Cataloging-in-Publication Data
Acampora, Christina L.
  Marketing chiropractic to medical practices / by Christina L. Acampora.
     p. ; cm.
  Includes bibliographical references and index.
  ISBN-13: 978-0-7637-5194-4 (pbk.)
  ISBN-10: 0-7637-5194-4 (pbk.)
  1. Chiropractic--Practice. 2. Chiropractic--Marketing. I. Title.
  [DNLM: 1. Chiropractic--organization & administration. 2. Marketing of Health Services--methods.
WB 905.7 A168m 2009]
  RZ232.2.A33 2009
  615.5'34068--dc22
                                             2008008858

6048

Production Credits
Publisher: David Cella
Acquisitions Editor: Kristine Johnson
Editorial Assistant: Maro Asadoorian
Production Director: Amy Rose
Senior Production Editor: Renée Sekerak
Production Assistant: Julia Waugaman
Associate Marketing Manager: Lisa Gordon
Manufacturing and Inventory Control Supervisor: Amy Bacus
Cover Design: Anne Spencer
Composition: Arlene Apone
Text Printing and Binding: Malloy, Inc.
Cover Printing: Malloy, Inc.

Printed in the United States of America
12 11 10 09 08   10 9 8 7 6 5 4 3 2 1

Dedication

Without the dedication, support, and encouragement of my family, this book would not have been possible. I am truly grateful to my husband, Steve, who did more than his fair share of the bath and bedtime routine while this text was being written. To my son, Weston, who is so supportive and proud that his Mom wrote a book, and to my daughter, Carly, who often toddled into my lap to "work on the 'puter" with me.

This book is also dedicated to the 60,000-plus chiropractors and upcoming graduates who make a daily impact on patient lives by offering an alternative, efficacious, and holistic choice of health care. May your passion and dedication shine through to the medical community.

Contents

A Note from the Author

This text has been a long time coming, not just because it has been a part of my life for the past five years, but also because it is the first sales and marketing book dedicated solely to the chiropractic profession.

It is important that you, the reader, understand what is and what is not included in this book. Because this book is dedicated to improving the relationship between the medical and chiropractic communities, it is therefore dedicated to improving public relations between our industry and the patients in need of our services who might not otherwise seek our care.

Many chiropractors resist or do not like to use the term *sales*, so for this reason, when possible throughout the book, I refer to this process as "promoting." The fact is, sales is as much promoting as promoting is sales. Sales is not analogous to slimy, sneaky, unethical, pushy, or any other action that has negative connotations like those associated with salesmanship. I know many ethical and well-respected salespersons in several different industries who are trusted by the people to whom they are selling. With this in mind, I present a sales method in this text that is conversational without being a sales pitch, and that is completely devoid of any type of pushy or obnoxious sales component.

Many of you might wonder why I am not promoting certain aspects of the chiropractic philosophy, but rather am emphasizing the success of manipulation and chiropractic management of neuromuscular conditions related to the lower back and neck. The answer is simple and straightforward: market research and common sense.

Market research discussed in this text examines what doctors are willing to hear about. As you will soon read, the medical community objects to the terminology chiropractors frequently use. However, chiropractic research is strong and accepted when it comes to the treatment of lower back pain, cervical pain, and headaches.

The common sense aspect comes into play through simple observation. Forcing ourselves onto the medical profession by educating the public about the vertebral subluxation process and proclaiming our ability to treat non-neuromuscular conditions have previously been met with significant opposition and further resistance by the medical community and many consumers.

To begin our integration with the medical community, we must embrace the trend of evidence-based chiropractic and use it to educate physicians on the effects of manipulation and chiropractic management of those conditions we can treat as supported in scientific journals. There is no reason why an approach such as the one used in this text that calls upon empirical research won't be readily accepted by the medical profession.

We are knocking on the medical profession's door. We can have it slammed in our face by promoting vertebral subluxation complex and lifetime care, or we can start providing the information the medical community responds to—such as how manipulation is an effective treatment for neuromuscular conditions. I can promise you that this book is not an antimedication or antisurgery campaign. It promotes other techniques that are competitive where the research allows them to be—but that is a part of the sales process, and I invite our competitors to try to refute what the research shows.

I invite your comments, questions, and promotional stories as we attempt to bridge this gap that has existed for too long between the medical and chiropractic communities.

Good selling!

Christina Acampora, DC

Acknowledgments

There are many phases of writing a book and many people to thank and acknowledge at each point for their input and advice.

I wish to acknowledge my publisher, Jones and Bartlett, who took a chance on this first-of-its-kind book for the chiropractic industry. Their editorial, marketing, and production teams have ensured that a quality text is presented to the chiropractic industry. A special acknowledgment goes to Dave Cella and Lisa Gordon for their guidance and extreme patience throughout the process. Thank you to the multidisciplinary reviewers, both chiropractic and allopathic, whose critique and input have helped this text evolve into its present form.

In the course of writing this book, I reached out to many chiropractic organizations and businesses to locate and verify the material and research included in this text. Their help and assistance identified key reports and viewpoints presented in this text. Their dedication and passion to protect and serve the chiropractic industry are evident.

Finally, I wish to acknowledge the many friends and family members who offered encouragement and support as I worked to complete this text. Special thanks to my parents, my in-laws, and my many "shire" and "cali" friends for your constant encouragement and support.

Chapter 1

Introduction

D o chiropractors need to market themselves personally to the medical community? The answer is a resounding yes! Specialists have many reasons to promote their services. All healthcare professionals, most notably specialists such as ophthalmologists, orthopedic surgeons, and neurologists, find themselves competing for market share as they also struggle to cope with shrinking healthcare reimbursements. All healthcare providers need referrals from physicians such as internists, osteopaths, and family practice doctors, and these doctors would like to know the types of services the specialists to whom they refer their patients perform.

Not too long ago my son needed a specialist referral, and our pediatrician strongly recommended a specific doctor, stating "I really recommend this doctor because I know what his examination and treatment protocols are." I took my son to this specialist because my pediatrician endorsed him so that I had immediate trust in his capabilities. Also, I knew that the specialist and my son's pediatrician would work together because they already had a professional relationship. This is the type of referral and endorsement you want physicians to give for your services as a chiropractor, and this textbook will show you how to get that.

Chiropractors are specialists in the treatment of neuromuscular conditions. Of all specialists, the chiropractic industry, especially, must also overcome a public relations issue. Consider the following issue. Manipulation has been proved to be safe and effective for treating several neuromuscular conditions, so other healthcare professionals such as physical therapists consider manipulation a therapeutic option and incorporate it into their educational programs. The physical therapy industry has proclaimed that it will be specialists in impairments and disabilities related to movement by 2020; it is a foregone conclusion that physical therapists will incorporate the use of manipulation in treating neuromuscular conditions. This shows that research on manipulation has opened doors for manipulation but not necessarily for chiropractors, who continue to stand outside of the medical circle. Physical therapists are already well incorporated in the inner circle of the healthcare arena and would be more than happy to introduce the use of manipulation to physicians. Where will that leave the chiropractic industry and the opportunity to increase our market share?

For chiropractors, there could not be a better time to educate physicians on manipulation. Baby boomers are aging, and it has been well documented that the cost of health care is a primary concern for those approaching retirement. Baby boomers and other healthcare consumers are interested in health care that provides an alternative to medication and surgery.

In addition to consumer demand, in March 2007 the American Heart Association (AHA) released a serious warning for those at risk of or who have heart disease to be cautious with their use of nonsteroidal anti-inflammatory drugs (NSAIDs).[1] The AHA also recommended that physicians use less invasive treatments when initiating patient care. This warning came as a result of increased risk of death or stroke for patients with long-term use of this class of drug. Those who primarily use NSAIDs on a chronic basis are those with chronic neuromuscular conditions. For example, chronic lower back pain sufferers make up the bulk of those with neuromuscular conditions who might use NSAIDs. Clearly, the purpose of revised treatment guidelines for chronic pain is not to favor one specialty or treatment over another. The purpose is to list choices suitable for use as alternatives to NSAIDs. Noticeably absent in the AHA guidelines is any mention of manipulation and chiropractic care. But it makes sense that the holistic treatment approach of chiropractors who use manipulation, exercise, and physical therapy, and who also promote patient self-reliance would be *the* most reasonable substitute for NSAIDs. Chiropractic care might also be the least invasive and safest starting point for any patient with a chronic neuromuscular condition.

The AHA publishes the prestigious scientific journal *Stroke*. Research on the safety of manipulation has been reported in *Stroke*. One such research report by Deanna Rothwell is illustrated in this text for you. The authors note the relative safety of and rarity of strokes related to manipulation, but even this report and other research articles like it aren't enough to gain chiropractic or manipulation a place on the list of viable alternatives to medications. Some medical doctors are concerned with the safety of medication and its demand by consumers. These doctors are open to learning about complementary alternative care.

We in the chiropractic industry can't be passive-aggressive. Our industry has the research to support the fact that chiropractors are effective both in terms of treatment outcomes and treatment costs as well as safety. Research supports our industry's stance that we deserve a rightful place in the inner circle of health care. Research provides you with a tool to open the door. We as a profession can't get exasperated every time we are not mentioned as a treatment option for chronic back pain and other neuromuscular-skeletal

(NMS) conditions. We have to speak up and educate physicians one by one on where and when to use chiropractic services and what steps they can take to provide the most efficient and safest care. We need to create demand at the ground level.

So far, physical therapy and medications have been mentioned as competitors, but so is any type of holistic healthcare provider, such as an acupuncturist. In an ideal world, every discipline, be it complementary or allopathic, would work together as a team and provide options for our patients. The idea of one "right" or "universal" provider for every patient doesn't exist, especially because consumer demand is beginning to shape the new frontier of health care. As such, health care has become competitive. When you educate physicians about chiropractic care, you must point out how you and the chiropractic profession stand out from the competition. The positive findings in the research on manipulation extend into specific data on how manipulation compares to medications, acupuncture, physical therapy, exercise, and management by medical professionals for back and neck pain. In addition, the cost data illustrate that chiropractors can offer treatments that are more cost effective in treating back pain and that subsequently reduce the costs of medication usage, hospitalization, and lumbar surgeries while decreasing days on disability and missed work. Chiropractors have the competitive edge for treating neuromuscular conditions and can match the demand of consumers for less invasive and more holistic health care.

Seeking medical referrals is not a new concept. It has long been desirable to secure a solid referral source and create a positive relationship with physicians. To date marketing to the medical world has largely been done on paper. However, why should a doctor "meet" you and review your research on paper? Is it reasonable to think that a doctor will receive a marketing letter from you and reciprocate with a phone call and patient referrals? Maybe, if you are lucky enough to pick the right doctor. There are not too many of these doctors yet, and a lot of marketing letters are sent to the trash bin. Marketing to medical doctors is most successful when done in person, whatever your industry.

This is a multipurpose text. It seeks to bridge the gap between the medical and chiropractic communities. It seeks to improve chiropractic practitioners' quality of life by providing a professional marketing campaign that is both cost effective and can be done with integrity. It seeks to tap into chiropractors' most untapped new patient source. By empowering chiropractors by providing the tools to make them more effective in marketing, this book can help chiropractors understand how to take a conversational sales approach to state and local politicians, too. Doctors of chiropractic are passionate about their profession, and this passion makes for persuasive promotional efforts that can help restore the public perception of chiropractors, not only in the medical community but also for healthcare consumers. Medical perception in the past has negatively focused on the chiropractic industry's lack of scientific validity and associated claims believed to dupe the public into believing chiropractors could cure such diseases as cancer. To some effect, the medical community still feels that if they send a patient to a chiropractor, more than just a back complaint will be addressed. This leads doctors to be concerned that their patients will receive unsubstantiated and unnecessary care.

There is no better time to step up and claim our fair market share. It is time to introduce ourselves into the inner circle of health care and forge relationships with medical professionals. This book is devoted to showing you how.

The Chiropractic Quality of Life

Practitioners may feel that they must choose between two paths—
the noble road to mediocrity, and the shameful one to riches.
—Ronald Feise, DC, *The Path of Professionalism*

You can imagine a balancing scale that measures the quality of life for chiropractors. On one side of the scale are patients and their treatment successes, winning a managed care battle, looking at the next day's schedule and seeing that you are fully booked. The other side of the scale holds issues of income versus debt, practice instability, losing managed care battles (income), and looking ahead one week in the schedule and seeing far too many openings.

Being a chiropractor can be emotionally exhilarating as well as exhausting; there are many factors that affect quality of life.

On the one hand, most chiropractors I know want to be involved in a helping industry; many know someone who has been helped tremendously by chiropractic manipulation, and this makes them want to participate. Chiropractors are fortunate in that they can take a new patient from diagnosis through treatment and to pain resolution usually without referring the patient to an outside facility. (Many other specialties don't have this advantage. They may provide a diagnosis and then refer out, or they might have a patient referred in only so that they can provide treatment, and then they send the patient away, never to see him or her again.) Chiropractors get to know their patients and can treat them for a variety of injuries and flare-ups. (Medical doctors to some degree treat the same patients over the years, but their relationships with patients are different because of shorter office visits, a non hands-on approach, and the singularity of the office visits needed to treat the patients' conditions.) Chiropractors reap the personal and professional rewards of watching a desperate and irritable patient respond to chiropractic management and improve with care. Some patients even reach a point they didn't think was possible. Patients who are helped by chiropractic care make up the positive side of a practitioner's professional quality of life.

There is, of course, a flip side to the chiropractic career. Chiropractors practice in relative isolation from the medical world. Not many chiropractors rave about financial success, and none can say that they have found the true secret to gaining new patient referrals because truly there is no guarantee. Like for any business, marketing is a constant and permanent requirement. The trick is to make it enjoyable, consistent, and affordable. These obstacles, coupled with the isolation resulting from participating outside of the health-care arena, promote a lack of professional self-esteem for chiropractors. The scale might not ever be fully or perfectly balanced, and over the years, if esteem begins to drop, due to the constant struggle to keep a balanced scale, a more complacent and helpless state can take over. Having to rejuvenate yourself over and over again is demoralizing.

The chiropractic quality of life is an important issue for our national organizations to address. It is well recognized that being outcasts in health care is unhealthy for our industry, politically and in the managed care spectrum, unhealthy regarding our political clout, and unhealthy for our patients. Chapter 12 touches briefly on how to take the promotional approach outlined in this text and apply it to your local and state politicians. A frontline army of practicing chiropractors educating politicians as well as medical doctors could significantly support the efforts of our state and national organizations.

Chiropractors take a lot of criticism. We are criticized at the outset because we don't need a 4-year undergraduate degree to enter chiropractic college. However, the prerequisites for chiropracty consist of upperclassman units of biological sciences. After graduating from chiropractic college, chiropractors are criticized for not being "real doctors," yet the Doctor of Chiropractic degree is considered a "First Professional Degree." Other examples of First Professional Degrees are the degrees of lawyers, veterinarians, and, yes, medical doctors.

Chiropractors face challenges in employment. You might expect that the dedication of obtaining a higher-education degree would at least provide some financial stability and career opportunities. For most chiropractors, it means self-employment, internal competition, and high student loans, which you will see make up the bulk of all health-related student loan defaults.

The clinical experience of many chiropractors offers them a first look at the world of sole proprietorship because much of the responsibility of finding patients rests with the student. Once graduated, new chiropractors rarely find an employed position, except maybe as an "exam" doctor for a busy practice. The odds that this will turn into a true opportunity to manage and treat patients are slim. Doctors who land in a busy practice tend to hop around from one practice to another until they can afford to be out on their own. However, practicing in this manner makes stability harder to attain because every time they jump practices, they lose a percentage of their patients, making the achievement of stability difficult.

The Long Road to Practice Stability

Upon graduating, most chiropractors have two jobs. One, often unrelated to chiropractic, provides an income and pays the rent; the other is typically as an independent contractor and provides a place to treat patients. Independent contractor positions can be—and for the most part are—frustrating. Rather than encouraging a long-term working relationship between doctors, they tend to encourage an independent contractor to build up his or her practice enough to leave and start a new practice. This is a reflection on the motivation of the clinic owner, who is trying to cover overhead and limit outgoing expenses. The independent contractor provides some stability for even the more established chiropractors.

Some chiropractors break free of contract positions by purchasing an existing practice, which usually adds a business loan to a student loan. This was my preferred route after 4 years and two difficult attempts at sole proprietorships. The practice I purchased was built on a maintenance care concept and structure. It didn't matter if the patient was a healthy 20-year-old college student with a small "crick" in her neck caused by a bad night's sleep or a 40-year-old sedentary, overweight patient with recurrent bouts of moderate to severe lower back pain. Both would be prescribed treatment 3 times a week for 3 weeks, 2 times a week for 4 weeks, 1 time a week for 4 to 6 weeks, and so on. The patients' response to care did not alter the treatment program unless, of course, patients needed more care or a referral for further diagnostic procedures. My mistake in picking this practice was that I don't ascribe to this philosophy, but the practice was one of only a few available practices in my geographic area. I thought it would give me enough of a base to support myself to practice chiropractic 100 percent and escape a bad sole proprietorship and my second job as a corporate administrative assistant. All said, it met this goal but introduced the seesaw that would stay with me to varying degrees for the next 7 years: There would be great months of high practice stats followed by crushing lows. If I let my marketing guard down for even a few weeks, it resulted in a downward trend.

Being the clinic owner and managing sole proprietorships is also difficult because a lot of time and support is provided to the proprietor as they grow their business. In the growth phase, there was not much income for me as the business owner; and then when the income would become stable, the sole proprietor would leave to form their own clinic.

Although subletting space can help offset some of the overhead of business ownership, it does not eliminate the pressures of running and building a practice. For example, I still had to bring in an income of my own because, with 4 years of practice under my belt, I was finally living purely off the profits of my practice. What I found missing was a stable income, the ability to purchase a home rather than rent, and the ability to take luxury vacations. I entered my thirties with an average surviving practice that had its share of greatness. What I and many other chiropractors lacked was a 401(k), quality medical/dental/optometry insurance, vacation pay, sick pay, and so on. Meanwhile, my friends who graduated from college and walked into employed positions were buying new cars, talking 401(k) planning, and taking vacations to Hawaii. I never took a sick day. I couldn't—doing so meant canceling patients, which meant losing income and still having to pay my staff. Taking a vacation for longer than an extended weekend simply wasn't an option. Patients in pain won't wait for you to return; they'll go somewhere else. Some will return to you; some won't.

Shortly after I turned 30 years old, I became pregnant with my first child. I had to consider maternity leave. I must admit that this was when the challenge of practice first became an emotional chore. I had been in practice for the magical number of 5 years, yet I did not have the financial security of many of my nonchiropractor friends and neither did I have their perk of maternity leave. The major concern was to find an affordable solution to keep my patients happy in my absence. Fortunately, my colleague who also rented space traded services: I would do both our billing and collections from home, and she would treat my patients until I returned. This arrangement allowed me to take maternity leave while providing the best coverage for my patients. While my son slept, I did not rest; instead, I worked. I entered maternity leave with no paid time off and the responsibility of running the administrative side of the business from my home. The pressures of making sure rent, malpractice insurance, and all of the other bills were paid continued. The fact that my student loans were continuing to accrue interest and my payments made no dent in the overall balance caused me to begin questioning my career path. When I returned to practice, I went back more tired and stressed than when I left. My associate had done a great job, but I was now entering my sixth year of business on little rest, and my professional satisfaction was quickly waning. I had been in the field for 6 years and had no stability despite running my business by the books as I was taught to do. The constant worry about new patients and how many patients I saw each week was no longer fun; it was fatiguing and demoralizing.

My practice was located on a busy street near medical office buildings. I often wondered how I could get the nearby doctors to refer their back pain patients to my office. I knew there were many patients in need of my services, and I had room in my books to take them. I also felt that after 6 long years I was ready to move from average practice stats to strong practice stats and start earning the income that I felt might actually pay off my student loans!

Financial Quality of Life

As a profession, chiropractors have persevered against medical bias. We have only just wedged our way into mainstream health care despite the lack of our specialty's own internal identity. The efficacy of manipulation has secured it a place in managed care; it has even earned chiropractors the right to offer services within the Veterans Administration (VA) system, and impressively it has helped create the need at the government level for the National Center for Complementary and Alternative Medicine (NCCAM). This is truly remarkable forward motion, yet only a few chiropractors do well enough to carve out a living of any speakable means because the field medical doctors continue to be unaware of the benefits of chiropractic and continue to have a misguided concept of the value chiropractors bring for back pain patients. It is frustrating that chiropractors have documented the most research to validate the efficacy of manipulation compared to many other common procedures used to deal with the billion-dollar lower back pain health issue. Chiropractors are the most logical type of specialist to begin treatment for a patient with back pain because of the efficacy and safety of manipulation.

For chiropractors who have education loans, the "living" a chiropractor makes is oftentimes dismal. Staggering statistics on the U.S. Department of Health and Human Services Web site reveal that under the Health Education Assistance Loans program, chiropractors have a significant lead over other health professions for number of loan defaults.[2]

Of a total of 1,115 defaulted loans, 53 percent (594) of these are loans defaulted on by chiropractors. The next largest group is dentistry at 19 percent (212), followed by allopathic medicine (MDs) at 11 percent (127). This is mind numbing and of course more negative press for our profession. The U.S. Department of Health and Human Services Web site[2] lists the following default amounts:

Allopathic medicine	127 Defaults	$17,412,718 due
Dentistry	212 Defaults	$36,356,958 due
Chiropractic	594 Defaults	$65,545,188 due

You can divide the balance due by the number of defaults for each profession to get the following amounts for average per-person loan amounts:

Allopathic medicine	$137,108
Dentistry	$171,495
Chiropractic	$110,345

Chiropractors have the lowest average loan default amount but the highest rate of defaults, a staggering 53 percent. We cannot entirely blame this default rate on self-employment because dentists are also mainly self-employed, and dentists tend to have a higher loan average and higher overhead resulting from the costs of dental assistants and necessary equipment. The issue isn't that our schools cost more, and it isn't that our overhead is higher. So, what is the problem?

I cannot but help to think it has something to do with the fact that dentists are accepted in the medical community as specialists and have a strong identity, which translate into public acceptance and professional repute. In contrast, the inability to pay off student loans is yet a different aspect that brings down the chiropractor's quality of life and self-esteem. The average salaries of those in the dental and chiropractic professions are telling: Dentists average $100,000 annually while chiropractors average $52,719.[3] For the amount of training chiropractors gain and pay for as well as the responsibility inherent in their work, this is simply unacceptable. Certainly, a higher education and job responsibility should parlay into higher wages and salaries. When you enter chiropractic school and assume student loans, you expect eventually to make enough money to pay off these loans before retirement. But this doesn't appear to be the case for the chiropractic industry.

The percentage of chiropractors who earn a professional-level salary is small. The majority make enough to support themselves; however, the quality of life that this affords them is debatable. This majority make enough to survive, but many go without retirement planning. Chiropractors can bill $350,000 a year, but if managed care deducts to the "usual and customary" and your overhead is reflective of a busy practice, you may actually net less than someone billing $150,000 a year. With managed care cutting our fees, with the staggering high rates of loan defaults, and in comparison with other health-care professionals, it is clear that finding a way

Help with student loans is available to those who live in or will relocate to areas with shortages of primary care physicians. Contact the American Chiropractic Association (ACA) for more information. (http://www.acatoday.com) 703-276-8800 toward the financial satisfaction of chiropractors is critical, especially for those graduating with student loans.

Marketing to medical doctors to develop a more stable referral base uses our time and advertising budgets productively. This can help create a more stable financial outlook with a steady supply of new patients. This is not to suggest that your regular marketing can be given up entirely; it will always be a component of owning a business. But it does mean that we can use marketing for more direct gain; although some months may be better than others, your finances will be tremendously more stable, especially if you can market to and get referrals from more than one medical doctor.

With the burden of financial debt, in part from student loans coupled with decreasing insurance reimbursements and a smaller-than-ever cash-paying portion of patients, chiropractors are becoming desperate. Desperation and hopelessness can cause an increase in unethical behavior in the form of scheduling unnecessary office visits and engaging in insurance fraud. Fraud is a billion-dollar healthcare issue, especially for Medicare. Fraud has many faces and is an ugly part of the healthcare industry and every specialty.

Online there are plenty of articles about insurance fraud committed by chiropractors (just Google "insurance fraud AND chiropractors"). The media seems to feed off of stories of any chiropractor who does something wrong, whether it was done as a chiropractor or a citizen. Of all the healthcare professions, we must be extremely aware of our actions and how they appear to the public because we already must overcome years of bad press. It seems the press finds any unethical behavior by a chiropractor to be newsworthy.

Also, insurance companies are cracking down on chiropractors who bill for excessive or inappropriate testing, such as X-rays to look for subluxation, computerized inclinometry at every visit, surface electromyography, and thermography. Insurance companies have also started to crack down on maintenance care because there is no evidence to support whether it is cost effective or medically necessary. Recently, the Foundation for Chiropractic Education and Research (FCER) announced that it will conduct a study on maintenance care in the prevention of chronic neck pain.[4] The study is in its earliest phases, and the results are not yet in. Clearly, though, the study will focus on patients with a *history* of neck pain; even if the study concludes maintenance is favorable, it is not appropriate for chiropractors to use maintenance care to boost insurance reimbursement in the asymptomatic patient who has no history of recurrent neck pain.

Until now, there was no written guidance available for chiropractors to help themselves financially by learning how to market successfully to medical physicians; most of us attempted to try what few options there were. Currently, medical marketing for chiropractors represents an enormous untapped market.

Time to Make Some Life Changes

Disenchanted after 10 years of practice, I left the profession all together, and on the recommendation of a friend I pursued a job in pharmaceuticals. Securing a job in a pharmaceutical company proved to be a challenge with a chiropractic degree, but it was possible. I later returned to the chiropractic profession with the realization that, like most situations, things happen for a reason. In my case, leaving the chiropractic profession led to a job in pharmaceuticals, which then provided the sales and marketing answer addressed in this book: "How can chiropractors best integrate with the medical profession to secure medical referrals?"

I have traveled full circle, and I returned to the chiropractic profession because I knew I had stumbled on the answer. I was good at pharmaceutical sales, and my job was very similar to some components of a chiropractor's daily life. We sell or promote to our patients all day long by educating them on their condition and explaining the risks and benefits of the procedure we use to treat them. Selling pharmaceuticals is similar because pharmaceutical company representatives use research findings to educate healthcare providers on who and what conditions the medication is for; they sell against competitors by educating physicians about the benefits of their company's particular drug compared with competitors' products. The process is no different for chiropractic sales, just the research and the level of professionalism as well as the authority with which it is delivered.

This text demonstrates a sales process that provides you with the tools to improve your practice without spending a lot of money. It shows you how to hit the correct target audience: Patients who actually have back pain. It shows you how to stand up with confidence and promote chiropractic ethically and professionally to the medical world. This can open the door to the medical world's inner circle. In doing so, it ensures that our profession promotes itself cohesively and based on research, which offers a possible answer to chiropractic's internal identity crisis. By integrating with the medical profession and adding value to patient treatment options, we begin down the path to joining the healthcare circle and leave the chiropractor's isolated world behind. We can then take charge of our careers.

Chiropractic Marketing

Have you seen the lonely chiropractor standing in a mall kiosk holding a spinal subluxation measurement gizmo with shoppers walking clear around to avoid the kiosk? Perhaps you have even been that chiropractor. I continue to feel sorry for these practitioners, but I admire the fact that they are out there trying to sell their services. Although I have never tried it and can't speak about the success of it, I suspect that if it was a successful method of gaining a steady flow of new patients, there would be more buzz around it.

A lot of marketing ideas are available and vary in price and value, but none tap the substantial number of patients experiencing back pain. Many Web sites for chiropractors offer marketing ideas. Here are some that in 15 years haven't changed—they all target directly the consumer willing or desperate to see a chiropractor:

- *How to do a review of findings.* Typically, the advice is that you do not review the findings on the patient's first visit; rather, you hold the findings for a second visit, which adds a visit and more charges. This is unethical because unless you are waiting for results from a special study, you can provide the diagnosis for the patient at the end of the first visit. You can report the findings to patients without paying someone to put an unethical spin on the report.

- *How to optimize your office layout.* "Use a line of benches to optimize your office layout. Then, you can zip up and down the rows adjusting backs in an unpersonalized and unprivate manner." Again, I think this is poor advice. We are not mechanics delivering manipulation to machines. We are doctors who talk about and treat private health matters for patients, and patients deserve the respect of not having to be treated in public. Also, with the Health Insurance Portability and Accountability Act in effect, patient privacy is a necessity. A couple of treatment rooms, a waiting room, and a restroom can be an optimal office layout.

- *Guarantee they will grow your practice for over $100,000 a year.* Or "Double your practice." This is a common marketing campaign that every chiropractor has seen. If it sounds too good to be true, it probably is. Rather, try limiting your expenses by educating medical physicians about chiropractic services. You'll spend less money and modify the plan to fit your own needs and personalities.

- *Use your business card as a coupon.* "Write in an expiration date on the card to bring in clients." But what if the person does not have back pain before the coupon expires? The effort that this takes to get one patient could be spent on reaching out to a medical doctor for several patient referrals.

- *Have your staff ask for one referral from one patient a day.* Please don't; it is tacky and the patient may feel uncomfortable or think you are struggling. If you provide a good service and the patient has a friend in need, he or she will advocate your services without being asked to do so. Asking for referrals may make you look desperate.

- *Advertise your business on water bottles for a local race.* Although this is good public relations and may be worth it, I wonder how many people throw away the bottle before noticing you provided it for them? This sounds like an expensive strategy as a new patient marketing tool; as a community exposure or public relations campaign, it sounds more acceptable.

- *Meet new people every day and send them a thank-you note.* Although this might get your practice's name in front of people, it may also be perceived as strange by the recipient. Rather, strive to meet medical physicians and set up a meeting to educate them about chiropractic services. If you want to reach out to consumers, try inviting them to an educational talk, or provide them with your office brochure.

- *Sell chiropractic as an alternative to medicine, not alternative medicine.* We are not an alternative to medicine. This is perhaps one of the most alarming statements I have seen. This is outdated and old-fashioned advice. If firms that promote this advice did their research or paid attention to what the public wants, they might have noted the following publicity failure from an article in *Chiropractic & Osteopathy* before suggesting it to you and charging you for it.

> Should the chiropractic profession concern itself with what others think? It should, must and had certainly better do so as it is reliant upon its consumers for its existence. A profession is a public trust. The privileges accorded to a member of a profession are in direct exchange for professional members' service to the public. It is nonsensical to organize a profession in terms that are at odds with the public's perceptions of its interests unless a compelling and persuasive argument can be made that the public's perception is not in their best interest and is amenable to change. We maintain that there is no such argument. In fact, efforts to launch such a campaign have failed. For example, two recent public relations efforts have been attempted by chiropractic organizations. These efforts were preceded and followed by measure of the public attitudes toward the profession. In both cases, efforts to convince healthcare consumers about the role of subluxation in their lives backfired miserably. Not only were few persons encouraged to consult a chiropractor, but, the number of skeptics was increased and more respondents stated that they would seek a medical consultation first following the PR effort than before the campaign. The argument that the public can be persuaded to understand and accept the subluxation model of chiropractic has been tested and it has failed."[5]

- *Have a marketing plan.* If an organization is charging for this advice, it should explain what it means, of course, and what it should consist of.

- *Valpak coupon advertising.* I advertised with a coupon for a free examination for any new client. This was my most successful means of securing new patients. Some months I would receive 10 new patients the week the coupon hit; other times I wondered if Valpak had forgotten to include me! I could detect no rhyme or reason to the responses. However, I gave away my time and my services to draw new patients. It is common knowledge that if a service costs money, the consumer perceives value. If a service is given away, the consumer perceives the service is disposable. I knew that, but I needed new patients and this worked for me most of the time. I hope our profession is able to leave these types of marketing techniques in the past by becoming successfully integrated with the medical world.

- *Yellow Page ads.* Essentially, these ads are more affordable than monthly coupons if you keep the ad small, but you are competing with all your colleagues for a patient who blindly reaches for the yellow pages to look for a chiropractor. Most of our referrals come from our patients, so again, this is a hit-or-miss marketing campaign. I tried yellow page ads with horrible results, but I have colleagues who swear by them.

- *Health fairs. True* health fairs could be pricey, especially ones limited in the number of chiropractic booths available. I felt good about participating in these because they were health oriented and the participants were there to learn about health. These types of fairs are not frequently available; they are usually seasonal and as such are not a consistent source of new patients. For a chiropractor trying to integrate in a community and stay integrated in a community, health fairs are quality events and worth your time to have a presence.

- *Newsletters.* Newsletters are a great way to keep your practice base well informed and keep your name in the minds of past patients for when they might need your services again. With e-mail, it is more economical than ever to send newsletters and certainly easier. The added benefit of going green helps, too!

- *Wellness or spine classes.* These are a good way to get patients to your office, but I resented having to ask my patients for participant referrals and typically that is how you get people to come to these talks. It is a spin on asking your patients for referrals. As discussed in Chapter 12, "Other Promotional Opportunities," some improvements can be made for this type of public relations talk. Certainly, if you are having a talk, you should advertise in your office and note that nonpatients are also welcome.

- *Chamber of Commerce/Kiwanis/Rotary/networking groups, etc.* Joining these types of organizations is a nice way to integrate into a community. If you are a new business in town, joining is a great way to meet other business owners. The primary interest of some of these clubs is to have you invest time in the community on their behalf for local events; promoting your business is a secondary goal. Attend a few meetings of a specific group to determine if you want to join the group or just market to members, in which case you might approach the group to be a guest speaker rather than a member. If you approach them to be a guest speaker, be sure to read the final chapter of this text, which deals with different ideas for public speaking.

- *Medical marketing.* Without a doubt, marketing to medical doctors is the most direct way to find new patients with back pain. For example, my office was located on medical row in my town. I often watched the stream of cars driving up and down the street as patients visited their doctors. I could only imagine how many were seeking care for back pain. I attempted to market my services to medical doctors through form letters, letters of introduction, report of findings for common patients, and so on. None of this met with any success. I never gave up on this marketing because I was sure that it was the way to go and that eventually one of the doctors would take note. In 7 years, I never received a medical referral despite consistent medical marketing. There are some interesting research articles on the interactions between chiropractors and medical doctors. We examine these in Chapter 5 to gain a better insight on this target audience.

- *Personal injury attorneys.* I had success with this and developed a couple of great working relationships. Primarily, any patient whose attorney I didn't know became a marketing target for me, usually in the form of introductory lunches. Personal injury cases can be a solid source of cash, but the method of payment is not continuous, and it might be a year or two before you are actually paid.

- *Workers' compensation.* I befriended local claims adjustors and I advertised my services to local large companies. This topic is discussed further in Chapter 12, "Other Promotional Opportunities."

- *Specialty degrees.* Many specialty degrees and certifications add credibility and authority. If you have a diplomate in sports chiropractic, marketing chiropractic to sports physicians is a great choice. A chiropractor with a certification as a Qualified Medical Examiner will make more impact with local workers compensation claims adjustors and companies than a chiropractor without the certification.

    Furthering your education with a specialty degree can help you stand out among your peers as you compete for medical referrals.

So, this is the advice out there. It hasn't changed in a very long time, and chiropractors continue to miss the majority of back pain patients out there. I have no doubt from personal experience and from colleagues that some of these tactics have worked, but personally I know that we can improve upon these concepts.

One conventional tactic related to medical referrals is a service you can buy for $500 that provides you with the template for form letters you can send out on a routine basis to medical doctors. I have sold to medical doctors, and I can assure you that if you do not personally go into their offices and meet them to discuss the merits of chiropractic and which patients are best suited for chiropractic care, you will not be as productive as you could be. A form letter can't do what you can do in person. You have just spent at least 6 years in college, and I know you can send an introductory letter to a medical doctor without having to pay some firm $500 to illustrate the proper writing technique.

For a while I received a monthly letter from a psychologist. I received enough letters to recognize her name, but I threw away most of them without fully reading them; I never reached out to meet her. It got to the point that I never even opened the letters because I already knew what was inside. Was her marketing campaign successful? If her goal was name recognition, yes; if it was for me to give her referrals for patients who have coinciding back problems and psychological issues, no. Had she come in and introduced herself, she would have learned several things. One, at night I sublet my office to a psychologist to cover overhead, so I had an allegiance to and first-hand knowledge of this person. Second, the letter-sending psychologist needed to sell her services to me and put herself in my mind when I had a patient in front of me who would benefit from her services. For instance, she could point out the rate of depression accompanying chronic back conditions and the positive impact treating the emotional component could have on my treatment plans. Quite frankly, I would not send my patients to her just because she mailed out a good letter. I still didn't know her; I didn't even know what she looked like. A professional introduction goes a long way to helping other providers remember your name and making a good first impression. This psychologist wasted effort and money, when instead she could have come in to meet me, find out about my patients' needs, determine whether she could help with any of those needs, and educate me about how to use her services. Chiropractors can do the same thing with medical doctors. It may be more intimidating, but certainly it is more fruitful. Introductory letters aren't bad, but they aren't as effective as personal visits and it could take a couple of years to determine if letters generate any business. Meeting a doctor in person can provide immediate feedback.

To market my business, I did everything I could afford to do and knew to do—except recommend maintenance care. I simply could not recommend care for a patient with benefits that are unsubstantiated. The research supports my viewpoint.

Chiropractic Earnings

More recent salary and expense surveys report current self-reported practice statistics. The information in Figure 1–1 is taken from the *Chiropractic Economics* 10th, 9th, and 6th Annual Survey Salary and Expense Surveys.

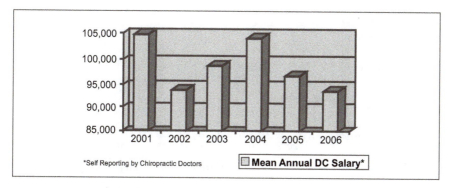

Figure 1–1   *Chiropractic economics information.*
Source: Adapted from *Chiropractic Economics.* Annual salary and expense surveys 10, 9, and 6.
Available at http://www.chiroeco.com/

Figure 1–1 illustrates the chiropractic industry as a whole, including the ebbs and flows of chiropractic income. The income for all of these years averages $98,642 with 4 of the 6 years showing earnings of less than $100,000. When you compare this average salary with the average defaulted student loan balance discussed earlier, which is $110,345, the financial quality of life of chiropractors becomes more clear. For example, for a 30-year loan at 6 percent interest, the monthly payment is roughly $660 for the average student loan amount. That is a large payment that can preclude many chiropractors from owning real estate or reinvesting in their business beyond covering monthly expenses. A chiropractor's average annual income just isn't enough, even if you are fortunate enough not to have a student loan.

Case in point is the following:

> When you closely look at the data, it's easy to conclude that chiropractors are working harder today—and earning less for their time. For example, according to the survey, in 2000, respondents said they saw on average 97 patients per week, and they had gross billings of $250K–$349K. This year, respondents said they see an average of 133 patients per week. Their median gross billings? The same as in 2000—$250K–$349K. In 1998, chiropractors reported paying themselves a salary of $131,200. That dropped to $76,100 in 2000, and has see-sawed ever since. This year's mean salary of $96,772 represents a decline of 7 percent from 2005. (Salaries of employees also showed a decline from 2005.)[6]

Chiropractors rely mostly on managed care for reimbursement; reductions in reimbursements have created the need for chiropractors to see more new patients, resulting in increased advertising overhead. The chart in Figure 1–2, which is taken from *Chiropractic Economics,* illustrates the climb in advertising costs.

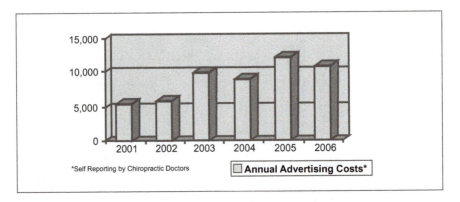

Figure 1–2 *Advertising costs.*
Source: Adapted from *Chiropractic Economics.* Annual salary and expense surveys 10, 9, and 6.
Available at http://www.chiroeco.com/

The financial seesaw can and does lead to desperation and unethical behavior, such as *upcharging*. This is when practitioners report the amount of time spent with patients as higher than the actual amount spent so that insurance companies must reimburse them at a higher rate. If you opt to be a provider in a network, you agree to treat in-network patients the same as all other patients, regardless of the reimbursement you receive. Upcharging causes concern about errors, misdiagnosis, and the potential destruction of the hallmark of our profession: patient satisfaction. In addition, the Evaluation and Management (E/M) Codes provide that a certain amount of time was spent with the patient for the medical decision making required for each service. This type of discrepancy between actual time spent with a patient and an E/M Code that charges for more time is obviously both unethical and illegal. If you don't like the reimbursement rates of a particular provider, then opt out of the network at once; don't cheat the patients.

Professional and Collegiate Relations

As a pharmaceutical representative, I occasionally called on Stanford University. The relationship between the university hospital and the community physicians was very interesting. The local hospitals host Grand Rounds that take place in almost all the hospitals usually on a monthly basis at no charge during a lunch hour with sandwiches provided to eat during the lecture. They are open to all physicians whether or not they graduated from Stanford. Grand Rounds is an educational program that calls upon thought leaders and researchers to present a large variety of topics, such as the latest evidence on treatment options for various conditions including pharmacologic options, diagnostic procedures, and radiologic findings. The presentation may also be a case report on a series of patients and an overview of case presentations, diagnostic findings, and treatment results. The lecturers are sometimes from Stanford and often from other colleges throughout the nation. Grand Rounds are well attended, giving community physicians interested in the presentation topic access to thought leaders and time at the end of the lecture to ask questions. In smaller one-on-one settings, these types of consultations are referred to as curbside consults.

What I really like about the whole concept of Grand Rounds is that it provides a setting in which physicians can come together to gain insight on a topic or be brought up-to-date on current research. It is an opportunity for them to see colleagues and have access to thought leaders. Many of the presenters are local college professors, fostering collaboration between academia and field doctors. For instance, as the lecturers became more familiar with local physicians, they might ask a physician into the classroom to present an interesting case study of a patient. This brings real life into the classroom.

It would also be very desirable for the chiropractic colleges to leverage their own thought leaders and local medical physicians to present to the community in the same manner as Grand Rounds, to reach out to the medical doctors who might be interested in the latest research on manipulation. Chiropractors can look to their local hospitals for Grand Rounds–type topics and lectures that they find interesting. I look forward to the day that chiropractors are one of the specialists that regularly present on back pain at Grand Rounds.

If you live near a chiropractic college, the school can be a great resource for curbside consults, if the professors are willing. Colleges are also an affordable resource for patients without insurance who are in need of chiropractic care because colleges offer a lower cost of treatment. You can view this as a problem if you think the college will entice some of your patients away, but there are several benefits to developing relationships with local academic institutions. Enhancing postgraduate relations between chiropractic colleges and local chiropractors may improve the current rate of patient referrals from area chiropractors to colleges. Interns need to see patients to get real-world experience and true clinical practice. Enhancing relations between colleges and local clinics may also improve the opportunity for research. Community chiropractors who are more involved with the local chiropractic colleges will be more aware of the research done at the college and may be more likely to support the research program by referring specific patient types who meet the criteria of the research project. Grand Rounds and other community outreach efforts from chiropractic colleges provide an opportunity to educate local chiropractors on the current research being conducted in their community. Yet, until the majority of chiropractors are busy enough to refer out a patient, referral relations between colleges and chiropractors may not be much of a reality.

Many references in the literature by prominent chiropractic researchers, the NCCAM, and National Institutes of Health (NIH) cite the need to increase the quality and quantity of the research at the chiropractic college level. Doing so would certainly enhance public relations and add legitimacy to our profession. When I talk to doctors and present research, they oftentimes comment that they didn't know chiropractors practiced evidence-based chiropractic. Chiropractic colleges that conduct research would also benefit from medical referrals by extending their research needs to local medical physicians for improved patient recruiting. However, not until local medical physicians truly understand chiropractic care will this be achievable.

By developing professional relationships with colleges, we might also influence the opportunity to establish relationships with local medical schools to increase grant funding opportunities. These types of relationships are encouraged by grant funding requirements at the NIH and the Health Resources and Services Administration (HRSA).[7]

Referrals Between Chiropractors and Medical Professionals

In 2003, the University of California, San Francisco, Center for the Health Professions produced a document by Bram B. Briggance, PhD, the associate director of the Workforce Initiative at the Center for the Health Professions. He noted that chiropractors seem to work in relative isolation from other practitioners and health professionals.[8] When chiropractors were asked if they received referrals from other practitioners, 92 percent of surveyed chiropractors responded yes, yet the frequency was noted to be no more than 1 to 2 a month and most fell below an average of one or two a year to none at all. In fact, only 50–60 percent of medical doctors refer patients for chiropractic care. Chiropractors were also found to be equally reserved when it came to referrals, and most referrals made were to internists, orthopedic specialists, neurology specialists, and massage therapists.[9]

Another study published in the *Journal of Manipulative and Physiological Therapeutics* in 2001 stated that only 10 percent of general practitioners (GPs) refer patients to chiropractors.[10] Referral of patients was found to be significantly related to the GPs' perceived knowledge of chiropractic and positive opinions regarding their past communications with chiropractors.

If you ask a medical doctor about chiropractic care, you will find that most agree that chiropractic works for back conditions, but they will express concern about how chiropractors require patients to come back. A few medical doctors may even state that people should not have their necks adjusted because it isn't safe. The bottom line is that the medical world tolerates chiropractors but certainly hasn't embraced us because of misperceptions; ironically, these misperceptions were largely created by the chiropractic profession. For example, the medical world questions how effective manipulation can be if the patient is forever forced to return for care. Medical doctors question the costs of this care in a time when health care is no longer affordable and evidence-based research defines healthcare providers' identity. There is no empirical evidence that wellness care is effective, and it is not reimbursed by insurance. If chiropractors desire medical referrals, they should focus on a treat-and-release philosophy for most of their patients. No empirical research supports any other philosophy, and the cost of unnecessary maintenance care is simply too great for consumers.

Public and Medical Perceptions of Chiropractors

Despite the fact that chiropractors perform 90 percent of manipulations and clearly have the most in-depth training and continued clinical experience with which to perform manipulations compared with osteopaths, physiatrists, and physical therapists, we are still viewed with a skeptical eye.[11] If our trade tool (manipulation) is now becoming popular because of research that affirms its efficacy but our utilization by the public is only estimated at 17 percent, we have a public relations issue.[5]

If you ask the general public what a chiropractor does, the most likely answer is one centered around manipulation of the spine, often more crudely referred to as "neck or back cracking." Although this isn't the most accurate way to say it, at least they all recognize that chiropractors provide spinal treatments. If you ask medical doctors what chiropractors do, they will provide a similar answer but add a misinformed precautionary statement about safety. Most every person will indicate that patients must keep going back to receive treatment; some might comment that they love their chiropractor; *they see him every week!* However, a survey by the National Board of Chiropractic Examiners (NBCE) found that only 9.3 percent of patient visits were related to wellness/preventive care. The trend of using chiropractic for wellness is changing, but the perceptions about chiropractic practice have not yet caught up.[12]

Following is an excerpt from a *Consumer Reports* (CR) article that is indicative of the public perception of chiropractic:

> Alternative medicine is no longer truly alternative. A *Consumer Reports* survey of more than 34,000 readers reveals that many people have tried it, and more and more doctors are recommending it. Readers gave the highest marks to hands-on treatments,

which worked better than conventional treatments for conditions such as back pain and arthritis. Chiropractic was ranked ahead of all conventional treatments, including prescription drugs, by readers with back pain. (Readers said it also provided relief for neck pain, but neck manipulation can be risky and is not recommended by *CR*.) Deep-tissue massage was found to be especially effective in treating osteoarthritis and fibromyalgia. While readers suffering from back pain deemed acupuncture and acupressure less effective than chiropractic and massage, one-fourth of readers who had tried these therapies said they helped them feel much better. Of all the hands-on alternative therapies, acupuncture has the most scientific support.[13]

I deeply disagree with this assessment by CR on two major issues. First of all, patients seek different complementary and alternative medicine (CAM) providers for different reasons. If they are referring to back pain, manipulation has the most evidence-based support even over acupuncture. In fact, in Chapter 8 I review head-to-head data comparing manipulation to acupuncture and NSAIDs and conclude that manipulation is more efficacious for spinal mechanical conditions, especially in the long term. There is no contradictory research to refute this paper. Second, CR is not a scientific journal and neither does it have the authority or expertise to recommend or not recommend a treatment. Research to date has been unable to prove significant risk to be associated with manipulation.

Even patient satisfaction with chiropractic care is disputed by medical critics, who suggest that patients are more satisfied the longer they receive treatment because of the hands-on nature of chiropractic treatments. Might not patient satisfaction result from the efficacy of manipulation rather then because of its hands-on approach? Might not patient satisfaction for many chronic back pain patients result from finally seeking effective treatment on their own because they are frustrated with the lack of progress made on their pain by traditional medicine? A patient once came in to my practice who was large and gruff and extremely grumpy as a result of his constant pain. This patient had come to me as a last resort, forced to do so because his wife insisted. He told me straight out that he didn't think chiropractic would work for him. Manipulation was more effective and it didn't take long for me to change the grumpiness into happiness and patient satisfaction. Patients like this and many others are helped because manipulation works, not because chiropractors put their hands on them and sympathize with their rotten luck at having a bad back. Some medical doctors suggest that chiropractors treat outside of their expertise. However, a survey by the ACA indicates that NMS conditions make up 94 percent of the conditions treated by the average chiropractor.[1]

The discord between the medical and chiropractic professions is not lost on patients. Just as many do not tell a chiropractor what medication they are taking, many more neglect to inform their physicians that they use chiropractic care for fear of being told not to. In fact, some patients won't even mention a visit to a chiropractor to their spouse. I once had a patient ask me to avoid billing her insurance because she didn't want her husband to learn that she sought chiropractic care. I asked myself, Would patients really go to this level of deception if they did not truly realize a valid positive impact on their pain from a discredited specialty? Both chiropractic and allopathic providers must be very careful not to judge a patient's decision about appropriate care for his or her condition.

It is possible for the chiropractic profession to educate physicians about chiropractic, who will in turn educate patients about the fact that a chiropractor is the least invasive provider who can treat neuromuscular conditions and who specializes in administering manipulation, which has been found to be one of the most efficacious and safest treatments for conditions such as acute and chronic lower back and neck pain as well as some types of headaches. Unfortunately, despite the public's willingness to see chiropractors as spine specialists, chiropractors still see only an estimated 17 percent of patients who could benefit from chiropractic care.[5]

It is up to chiropractors to identify the treatments for which manipulation is indicated and to educate physicians on the benefits of chiropractic care, clearing up the misconceptions that continue to haunt the chiropractic community. Chiropractors can make the most impact if they present a unified front to promotional efforts. Referencing credible research is one method of providing the much-needed united identity.

Identity

Acceptance by the medical field does not need to mold our profession's identity. The research is doing that. Acceptance by the medical field does not justify our existence, but it does improve our self-esteem. As chiropractors, we have all had moments when we have proudly proclaimed, "I am a chiropractor." As time passes, we make the proclamation more quietly as we anticipate people's negative or suspicious or pity-filled responses. It shouldn't be this way. The empowerment of knowing the research that is presented in this book supports your services, knowing that your care is effective, and that you rightfully deserve a place in health care can provide a powerful sense of inner security. If a medical doctor doesn't like chiropractors, it shows that he or she is not aware of the best treatments for patients. Most likely, though, it isn't that doctors don't like chiropractors, it's that they just don't understand what we do.

It is time to evolve from what chiropractic once was and catch up to what it has become. To know what the chiropractic industry once was, we must look at our founding fathers, namely D.D. and B.J. Palmer. Chiropractic has been around 100 years. Some doctors of chiropractic still follow the original treatment philosophy and continue to insist that chiropractic is the answer for everyone and that everyone needs monthly adjustments. They will tell you that the body has innate intelligence if properly aligned and can ward off diseases such as mumps instead of relying on vaccinations. Chiropracty used to support these vitalistic unsubstantiated views. That has changed recently in chiropracty. It is evident from the numbers quoted earlier that wellness and maintenance treatment are but small fractions of a modern chiropractor's practice.

One of my favorite journal articles discusses the identity crisis of chiropractic and its place in the healthcare system. It was published in July 2005 in *Chiropractic & Osteopathy* and titled "Chiropractic as Spine Care: A Model for the Profession."[5] It is a must-read article if you haven't already. The authors offer an in-depth comparison of the chiropractic profession with the dental profession. This comparison is not a new one; however, the authors break it down in its importance to the chiropractic world. What makes the article all the more compelling is the fact that it is written by notable thought leaders in the chiropractic profession who are heavily involved in research and also four of whom work at American Specialty Health (ASH). ASH is one of the nation's leading complementary healthcare benefits organizations.[14]

It is logical to assume that these managed care chiropractors are trying to help out their professional community while working within the constraints of a managed care organization. This glimpse into their professional opinion should be taken seriously because they identify a model for the profession that will help integrate chiropractic care with the medical profession and improve the overall public image of chiropractic services. The solution they offer for the chiropractic identity crisis does not interfere with the self-identity of chiropractors, and it has every reason to be accepted by the medical profession. The following quote underscores the sense of urgency of why chiropractors need to educate the medical profession.

> It is always fashionable to speak of an issue or controversy as reaching a "crisis point," or of an organization or profession reaching a "crossroads" in its development. However such exhortations are often merely hyperbole. At the risk of committing this offense, we believe that the chiropractic profession today faces an exceptionally difficult set of challenges and, yes, a crisis. The nature of this crisis is the profession's continued inability to

define itself. The chiropractic profession, more than 100 years after its founding, does not project a definition of itself that is consistent, coherent or defensible. The healthcare system is increasingly intolerant of such ambiguity and uncertainty; an intolerance which will only intensify in the future.[5]

Our chiropractic representatives at ASH are concerned about our industry. Our thought leaders in research who produce some of the most compelling research substantiating the efficacy of chiropractic are concerned. The profession as a whole has yet to come together as a solid unit. First, we must figure out where we would like to fit in. Can we be mainstreamed with the medical world and still maintain our identity as holistic healers, and if so, how?

The answer is that we can start integrating with the medical community by promoting the research. As chiropractors we can promote the evidence and define ourselves as specialists for neuromuscular conditions. Emphasize the fact that we focus on wellness through education, exercise, and living a healthy lifestyle, which only follows consumer desires for emphasis to be placed on being healthy and not on being sick. We do not promote "wellness"-based or "maintenance" chiropractic visits or treatment plans. By educating physicians with the evidence, we bring legitimacy to the chiropractic profession, which improves medical relationships and public relations and legitimizes chiropractic once and for all. The responsibility for this type of public relations lies with our national organizations, chiropractic research, and each of us.

People have the right to think and believe what they want, but as health practitioners we have sworn to first do no harm. If a condition does not empirically show improvement with chiropractic care, as a professional we must accept it and move on. For example, the battle over whether to vaccinate or not has been fought already; doctors are strongly in favor of vaccinations. Chiropractors won't always like the outcome of the research, but this research shapes our role in the healthcare industry and allows us to be better healthcare providers for our patients.

I would like to share a story about my father. At 61 years of age my father began experiencing "memory lapses" and confusion. My mother described him as just "being out of it." The symptoms were transient but concerning enough to my mother that she took him to doctors, one of whom was new in town and highly regarded. In the small community where they live, there weren't many doctors. The remedy the new doctor devised was switching my father to a vegetarian diet. This was not an appropriate recommendation based on any clinical findings this doctor had qualified; it was especially inappropriate for a man who was only 61 and loved to barbeque. When any doctor recommends a treatment, it must be something that a patient can actually implement. Becoming a vegetarian at 61 years of age was not realistic and neither did the doctor send my father to a nutritionist to learn how to be a well-balanced vegetarian. Although a more conservative approach to diet was in line, starting a vegetarian diet was a recommendation that was made not on medical science but by personal beliefs. This doctor was a 7th Day Adventist for whom vegetarianism reigns supreme. Needless to say, my father did not get the care he deserved, and managed care paid for a service that wasn't appropriate or competent. The clinical presentation of my father's condition, coupled with his wife's concern, should have dictated more tests. This doctor didn't even order bloodwork to look at his cholesterol prior to recommending the diet change. A couple of months went by and the attacks continued and worsened. My mom took my father to her nurse practitioner, who ordered the appropriate testing. The result: A sudden and surprise quintuple cardiac bypass. My father's heart was 90% blocked in several areas, 100% in another; the ambulance literally picked him up at the doctor's office where he had undergone an angiogram and whisked him off to another hospital for surgery. The moral is: Believe what you want to believe, but practice by the guidelines, and utilize appropriate clinical experience in combination with valid research. It takes only one experience for a person to form an opinion, and this relates to the opinion many medical doctors have of the chiropractic industry from past experiences with chiropractors who may not have based their treatments on science.

As the authors of "Chiropractic as Spine Care" point out, chiropractors are not "disease prevention specialists." Although some of us refuse to move away from this idea, more chiropractors identify with the authors on the following identity for the profession:

> *"Chiropractic as an NMS specialty, with particular emphasis on the spine"*
>
> *"Chiropractic as a portal of entry (POE) physician/provider"*
>
> *"Chiropractic as a willing and contributing part of the evidence-based healthcare (EBHC) movement"*
>
> *"Chiropractic as a fully integrated part of the healthcare system, rather than as an alternative and competing healthcare system"*[5]

Some key challenges for our profession that center around chiropractic identity can be found in a key paper produced by The Institute for Alternative Futures (IAF):

- In general, a relative lack of awareness on the part of the broader public of the value of chiropractors' services
- Focus-of-practice questions (whether and how far chiropractic should extend beyond back problems)
- Lack of professional solidarity

- Reimbursement restrictions
- Potential rise in competition from other types of practitioners[12]

In addition, this article also identifies where the future looks brightest:

- Continued growth in the evidence confirming manipulation's efficacy and cost-effectiveness
- Continued high support among patients
- Better integration into the wider healthcare system, including more referrals both to and from medical doctors[12]

Whereas other professions have altered their identity to conform to allopathic care demands, chiropractors remain devoted to manipulation. Chiropractors lead the interest in formulating research designs, which has been pivotal in proving the efficacy of manipulation and has led to managed care coverage and Agency for Health Care Policy and Research (AHCPR) and Department of Defense inclusion of chiropractic services. Research is what has been shaping us, and it is what will continue to shape us. Our identity has yet to be found internally, but research may just do it for us. As Dr. Scott Haldeman notes, "If chiropractors do not accept this change many will find themselves in a kind of culture shock as the demands to follow this pattern pick up momentum. It must be realized that scientific research is forming the basis of the theories that direct further research and which therefore direct clinical practice."[15]

The World Federation of Chiropractic (WFC) offers the following definition of chiropractic, which allows for us to be both holistic healthcare providers and musculoskeletal specialists:

> A health profession concerned with the diagnosis, treatment and prevention of mechanical disorders of the musculoskeletal system, and the effects of these disorders on the functions of the nervous system and general health. There is an emphasis on manual treatments including spinal adjustment and other joint and soft-tissue manipulation.[16]

Portal-of-Entry Provider versus Primary Care Provider

It is important to note that some researchers define our role in health care as a POE provider. Patients have direct access to POE provider services similar to the access they have to dentists and optometrists. The public thinks: Eyes → optometrist, teeth → dentist, and back → chiropractor; all else goes to the medical doctors. This arrangement does not diminish our importance in health care; rather, it identifies us as specialists.

Curtis Turchin provides another interesting perspective on chiropractors as primary care physicians. He brings up some very reasonable counters on why chiropractors should not be primary care providers:

- More time at the college level studying microbiology and pathology, which decreases the available time to study biomechanics and adjustment procedures
- Increased malpractice rates
- Oversupply of specialists and increasing number of nurse practitioners and physician assistants to fill the void of any shortage of primary care doctors[17]

One other specialty is entering POE provider status and that is physical therapy. It is estimated that only 12–17% of Americans with back pain visit chiropractors of the 75% who could likely benefit.[5] The public either recognizes us or they don't. For those who visit us, it is a nice relationship; for those who don't, there is a lack of understanding that has not been improved upon. We need the medical profession to understand and help us to legitimize our services to the 83% of the back pain population not currently seeking our services. This new competition from physical therapists should make the sense of urgency to act one of your highest priorities. I discuss this more in Chapter 11, "Introduction to Competitive Selling."

A POE is necessary to control costs. Patients who seek chiropractic care on their own don't need a doctor to confirm that they have back pain, and it isn't convenient or cost-effective to see an MD for a referral for chiropractic care. Requiring a gatekeeper for back pain patients will only compound the financial impact back pain has on health care, especially when NSAIDs for certain subgroups are no longer recommended as first-line agents for certain populations, and especially when most MDs refer out their chronic back pain patients. Finally, there is no danger in having a chiropractor work up a patient because we are well trained to differentially diagnose neuromuscular back pain and back pain of a referred and potentially dangerous origin. This is supported by the US Government Accounting Office, which found that 60–90% of office-based diagnoses could be handled by non-MD professionals.[18, 19]

By opening access to all specialists, perhaps we free up time for the primary medical doctors to treat what they are best at, especially when a shortage of these medical doctors is anticipated in the near future. Medical doctors excel at listening to systematic complaints and working these up to either treat within their own office or to refer out. They have additional strengths in treating viral illnesses and administering medications such as antibiotics for these conditions. It is also fair to suggest they might like to be free of the referral paperwork and get back to doing what they do best, treating patients and not being administrative care providers. Obviously, managed care might have some objections for the free will of patients to seek care from specialists; however, most patients are reasonable and utilize the specialties appropriately. This, of course, comes in parallel with the emerging trend of consumer-driven care. "Many people (10%) are seeing multiple (second) providers for problems considered routine" and "the use of alternative providers and the fact that a great deal of such care is not disclosed suggest that the single point of primary care model is failing to meet the needs of many consumers."[19] Healthcare patients are now becoming savvy consumers. It is interesting to study the trends as baby boomers develop more health conditions and require more care. What will they demand?

Perhaps the best description of primary care comes from the NBCE: "Primary care is accessible, first-contact health care, without the necessity of a referral."[20] The NBCE survey also purports that our practice comprises treatment of musculoskeletal conditions and very rarely any other conditions.

Should Chiropractors Prescribe Medication?

There has been talk and desire by some chiropractors to be able to prescribe medication. For the purposes of promoting to allopathic providers and maintaining our identity as a nonpharmaceutical approach to treating musculoskeletal conditions, we are better off not to prescribe medication. As a previous pharmaceutical representative, I can promise you that chiropractors don't want the license to utilize medications. They would then be swamped with rep visits—just one drug class could bring as many as three to five pharmaceutical visits a week. More important, the ability to prescribe simply takes the focus off holistic health care, a niche that chiropractors excel at filling and one that is highly in demand.

It has also been noted that osteopaths who are primary care physicians are less likely to perform manipulations and spend more time doing primary care activities. I like the idea of maintaining our identity as holistic (nonthreatening and noninvasive) healthcare providers. It is certainly trendy in light of all the recent drug warnings. Plus, by sending our patients to MDs/DOs, we form relationships and create the back-and-forth referral system that allows us to truly integrate with them. Doctors are in business too and do not want to send their patients out the door. Sending patients who need medications to doctors allows us an opportunity to reciprocate the referral and maintain a professional interactive team relationship for the benefit of the patient without the headaches or the distractions of prescribing drugs.

The Competition

An entire chapter (Chapter 11) is dedicated to describing the competition, examining their strengths and how manipulation or chiropractic care compares in the treatment of neuromuscular conditions. Manipulation has enjoyed successful research, and many providers who are interested in physical medicine are picking it up as part of their treatment protocol. This provides a very real threat to the chiropractic industry. Chiropractors have not yet successfully integrated with medical physicians, whereas many of our competitors have. These competitors, such as physical therapists, will have a very easy time adapting manipulation to their treatment protocols and utilizing these protocols to educate physicians on their services. Aside from already being accepted by medical physicians, the adaptation of manipulation into the physical therapist's repertoire, their proactive movement toward POE providers, and their proclamation to be specialists by 2020, physical therapists also promote to medical physicians. In fact, their national organization provides Stark Laws specifically to ensure that their members promote properly to physicians. If chiropractors don't begin talking to physicians to educate them on manipulation, it is a certainty that our competitors will. Chiropractors have endured years of bias, and it would be devastating for another industry to promote manipulation in our place. The need for chiropractors to promote themselves is an urgent issue.

Baby Boomers

Baby boomers have been described as those born between 1946 and 1964. Their population totals 76 million, and they represent 28% of the American population today.[21] This is compared to Generation X (those born between 1968 and 1979) who total only 41 million. Baby boomers represent a unique and important population boom for chiropractors. They are an active, intelligent population in true need of musculoskeletal treatment and who will not simply be told what to do but who will research it themselves. Update your knowledge on golf-related injuries and be prepared to answer questions because this educated population will want to know the specifics! This generation wants care that is focused on maintaining activity levels and that is holistic and cost-effective.

Baby boomers are aging and have more aches and pains that cause them to seek care. Americans in their early to mid-50s report poorer health, more pain, and more trouble doing everyday physical tasks than their older peers reported at the same age in years past, according to the nonprofit National

Bureau of Economic Research.[22] As part of an abstract narrative for a current research project, Dr. Meeker notes that lower back pain in the elderly has a prevalence ranging from 13–49%.[23] Baby boomers will be sure to increase demand for therapies that improve their quality of life.[12]

A study, supported by the National Institute on Aging, a component of NIH, showed the following:

- The two younger groups (born in 1942–1947 and in 1948–1953) were less likely than the oldest group (born in 1936–1941) to have said their health was "excellent or very good" at 51 to 56 years of age.

- The youngest group reported having more pain, chronic health conditions, and drinking and psychiatric problems than people who were the same age 12 years earlier.

- Compared with the oldest group, the youngest group was more likely to have reported difficulty in walking, climbing steps, getting up from a chair, kneeling, or crouching, and doing other normal daily physical tasks.[24]

- "This new analysis provides some initial data raising the question of whether today's preretirees could reach retirement age in worse shape than their predecessors, with individuals potentially in poorer health than current retirees and possibly increasing healthcare costs for society."[24]

- "Researchers and policymakers are vitally interested in whether this trend will continue, accelerate, or decelerate with the retirement of the baby boom, a critically important concern in planning for health, housing, and other needs for this wave of retirees, who begin to turn 65 in 2011."[24]

On October 23, 2006, *Newsweek* published an article on baby boomers that discusses housing requirements, which interestingly parlays into community environments. Baby boomers are setting the demand for high-quality active living setting housing development opportunities focused on amenities for Pilates, home offices, fitness equipment, swimming pools, yoga, core training, adventure programming (whitewater rafting and skydiving), golf, and educational programs.[25] So much for bingo and rocking chairs!

Because this generation is expected to live longer than previous generations, there is a real and valid concern regarding money, especially for health care. This generation has watched their parents age and witnessed the out-of-pocket expenses paid for medication. Take my grandmother, for example. She had only Medicare coverage and lived a modest and enjoyable retirement until she died at 94 years of age. She enjoyed relatively good health and took medication for only a couple of conditions: High cholesterol and glaucoma. However, her medication costs alone were more than $500 a month for only two conditions, which in the scheme of things were relatively minor. These costs are expected to rise.

Cost-effectiveness will be a major issue not only for insurance companies but also for the patient. The cost-effectiveness data for chiropractic care are extremely compelling, yet insurance companies continue to deny reimbursement for chiropractic doctors.

Promoting Ourselves

My career path has provided profound insight from a selling component and most recently as a consultant for a medical facility integrating a complementary healthcare branch. I have seen what works and what doesn't.

Researchers point out that many primary care providers are not interested in treating spinal pain,[26, 27] and more than two-thirds of GPs say they would be interested in receiving information about chiropractic.[26, 28]

The chiropractic profession has had the research results for a few years, yet no one knew how to utilize it. Take, for example, the AHCPR report[9] that illustrates efficacy for manipulation for acute lower back pain. The chiropractic profession certainly knew about it, but little was done to promote it to field physicians—the ones who prescribe care and referrals for millions of acute low back pain patients.

Many examples have followed, including another prime opportunity in February 2007 when the AHA announced new clinical guidelines for chronic pain patients and the use of NSAIDs. It is a fact that certain populations of patients who are at risk of or have heart disease or stroke should use conservative care rather than NSAIDs as a first line of defense. The ACA posted the warning on its Web site, but again no chiropractor sat in front of a doctor and promoted care for patients who were no longer able to use NSAIDs and who suffered from lower back or neck pain.

We as field professionals have done nothing with this bevy of positive information but sit idle and hope that some "aha" light switch will go on in the medical doctors' heads. The fact that this information came out and we as a profession, although thrilled, did nothing with it to improve our status within the medical profession or to take advantage of it as a selling tool is a hallmark and testament to our past marketing abilities.

In contrast, when I was in pharmaceuticals, had a new clinical guideline like the AHA warning been issued that would have positively affected the company's promotional efforts, we would have had a voicemail from the president or vice president of the company, a voicemail from our regional manager, a voicemail from our district manager, and a voicemail from our regional sales trainer outlining how to take this new news and incorporate it in our selling technique. This isn't an oversight on our profession's part but rather a lack of understanding of how to utilize tools such as these and promote them to medical doctors.

Our industry is dropping the "promotional" ball every time this type of advantage is released and we do nothing with it. Our field chiropractors who are actively promoting to medical doctors should have downloaded this warning and dropped it off at every office they were acquainted with. If I couldn't personally speak to the doctor, I would have a brief typed letter such as the following:

Dear Dr. Internist,

Today the American Heart Association issued warnings for patients at increased risk of heart attack or stroke who were taking NSAIDs for chronic pain. The study and the AHA recommend new treatment guidelines for these patients in which the new treatment algorithm should begin with noninvasive care.

As we have discussed in the past, chiropractic is a perfect solution because it utilizes a noninvasive and nonpharmaceutical approach for patients with back pain.

[*Cite a study that you have covered or a newer one that discusses chronic pain.*]

I hope this information is helpful to you, and I enclose the full report from the AHA for your review.

I am looking forward to our lunch meeting on January 30th.

Sincerely,

Christina Acampora, DC

From a promotional standpoint, we have enough research data to emphatically promote manipulation and chiropractic care for the lower back and neck regions as well as for headaches. These are the conditions for which care should be promoted first. This is not to say that chiropractors can't associate themselves with carpal tunnel or knee pain and so on. The research shows that we get most of our business from treating the neck and lower back. The research also illustrates that doctors have few options to offer these patients except medication and referrals. By starting with these strong cases for which it is appropriate to utilize chiropractic care, we can then build trust and rapport that will open the door to referrals for other conditions.

The bottom line from a promotional standpoint is to promote only research referenced in a peer-reviewed, notable journal and to not stretch the meaning of findings beyond which they were intended to relate. If you believe drugs are bad, immunizations are unnecessary, and chiropractic can cure asthma, stop and reevaluate the position you are putting the profession in when you promote these unsubstantiated claims to medical doctors. Asthma is a great example because many chiropractors believe that manipulation can decrease corticosteroid and beta blocker use. Empirical research simply does not support this yet. What has been published on asthma has mixed findings. Accept the fact that chiropractors are very good at treating back pain and be happy with that until further research proves otherwise. Eighty percent of Americans will experience back pain at some point; back pain is one of the top five reasons people see a physician. With only 17% of the back pain population visiting a chiropractor each year, imagine the business that is available. Start by promoting care we can prove to be effective. Doing so will help the profession's image, our acceptance, our identity, our popularity. From there recognition will hopefully flow to managed care and politicians. If the public demands chiropractic care, so will the government. This equates to more funding for research and more investigations into other conditions we know we can help.

The impact of chiropractic not being accepted in the healthcare arena is being felt. In a recent article, Dr. Robert Mootz, DC, cites, "More than one third of Americans report that they used alternative therapies within the previous year, with back pain and neck pain representing 2 of the top 3 reasons for doing so" followed quickly by this alarming stat: "Chiropractic now appears to lead the alternative care pack for having the largest decline in use, with a full 2.5% drop in its use in recent years."[29]

Included in Dr. Mootz's assessment is the accurate observation that chiropractors seem content to preserve the status quo. I contend we maintain it because we simply haven't had the tools to empower ourselves. As Dr. Mootz also points out, he believes that we will be embraced if we harness the science and use it to refine and improve what we do. This article substantiates the viewpoint I have already outlined in this chapter; that it is addressed by a prominent chiropractic figure should make it all the more persuasive.

We are the third largest healthcare industry and the public perception is that we are spine specialists, yet we are seldom recommended as a treatment option in any type of medical literature and we treat only 17% of the patients out there. In my local newspaper I came across an article similar to many others I have seen in the past. The article was titled "Treating Pains in Your Rear" and appeared in November 2006. The discussion focused on sacroiliac joint pain, yet no mention of chiropractic treatment was made! How can the third largest healthcare industry noted as spine specialists with evidence on their side not be mentioned as a treatment option? It is truly remarkable.

When chiropractors promote themselves, they have always promoted themselves as wellness and prevention doctors. This is true, and chiropractors are truly valued by their patients as a result. However, chiropractors are not the only health professionals who promote wellness. In 2006, I was diagnosed with hypothyroidism. In treating me, my GP was extremely health conscious and interested in proper nutrition, diet, and so on. He wasn't satisfied by relying on medication alone to reverse my condition. A second example comes from my father's care, which I described earlier. After his quintuple bypass, the hospital before discharging him had him meet with multiple personnel who covered the necessary changes in lifestyle he needed to make, including nutrition and exercise. The exercise program he and my mother were highly encouraged to participate in is truly impressive. The distinction I am trying to make is that allopathic providers are heavily invested in disease prevention and healthy living, and it would be a mistake to promote wellness as unique to chiropractic care when it is also a trend that allopathic care providers are also promoting. It would not be a mistake to reiterate that wellness in the form of lifestyle changes, diet, and exercise also exist in your practice and would complement the doctor's recommendations to his or her patients.

In 1998, the IAF recommended that the newfound interest in CAM be taken advantage of by providing integrative care and developing better interdisciplinary teams.[12] However, little progress has been made since that recommendation. It is most likely a result of a lack of understanding of how to integrate. The IAF supports that although chiropractors have high patient satisfaction, the broader public is indifferent or negative. A referral from a medical doctor to his or her patients for chiropractic care will no doubt have a heavy and positive influence on this public perception.

The Good, the Bad, and Evidence-Based Health Care

The Good: Research

An interesting story was told by Dr. Scott Haldeman.[15] At a pivotal time in his career, he was invited to participate in the first formal interaction between chiropractors and medical physicians. It was in the 1970s and the US Congress had asked the National Institute of Neurological Disorders and Stroke to organize a conference on spinal manipulation. When asked at the conference for all attendees to propose speakers and topics, only Haldeman submitted anything. As such, 80% of the conference included his topics and choice of speakers. It was as he said, "names he had only read about." Murray Goldstein of the National Institute of Neurological Diseases and Stroke would later conclude that there was insufficient research to either support or refute chiropractic intervention for back pain and other musculoskeletal disorders.[30] This conference jump-started research for the chiropractic profession particularly by the ACA, the International Chiropractors Association (ICA), and the FCER.

Federal acknowledgment in the 1970s provided the financial funding chiropractors needed to perform research. Importantly, this research went on to secure recommendations of the AHCPR and managed care as well as laid the foundation on which all current legitimacy is built upon. RAND Health in 2001 stated, "Today, chiropractors are the 3rd largest group of healthcare providers, after physicians and dentists, who treat patients directly."[31] It was also noted that people go to alternative medicine practitioners more often than they see primary care physicians. Nearly half of alternative medicine visits are to chiropractors. As a result of this success, substantial organizations have been founded by chiropractors or include chiropractors on their panels.

American Back Society

The American Back Society (ABS) was founded in Oakland, California, in 1982 as a nonprofit organization dedicated to providing an interdisciplinary forum for healthcare professionals and scientists interested in relieving pain and diminishing impairment through proper diagnosis and treatment of patients suffering from spinal pathology. The society is composed of orthopedic and neurological surgeons, osteopathic physicians, physical therapists, chiropractors, neurologists, psychiatrists, radiologists, rheumatologists, internists, occupational therapists, nurses, psychiatrists, and other healthcare professionals. There are currently 13 committees, composed of these specialties, whose goals are to further the quality of education and knowledge of the ABS membership and the healthcare community, with the ultimate goal of improving back care.[32]

Agency for Health Care Policy and Research

Between 1992 and 1996, the AHCPR (now the Agency for Healthcare Research and Quality) sponsored development of a series of 19 clinical practice guidelines.[9] In 1994, it released Clinical Practice Guideline No. 14: Acute Low Back Problems in Adults. Although this paper is frequently quoted in research, it is now considered to be outdated, and no other updates have since been provided. Although outdated, the importance it held for the chiropractic profession can't be overlooked. It was one of the premier inclusions of manipulation as a choice for managing lower back pain. That it was a government guideline for treating acute lower back pain makes it especially monumental. Its recommendations for lower back pain were as follows: "Manipulation (in place of medication or a shorter trial if combined with NSAIDs)" and

> **Manipulation,** defined as manual loading of the spine using short or long leverage methods, is safe and effective for patients in the first month of acute low back symptoms without radiculopathy. For patients with symptoms lasting longer than 1 month, manipulation is probably safe but its efficacy is unproven. If manipulation has not resulted in symptomatic and functional improvement after 4 weeks, it should be stopped and the patient reevaluated.[9]

National Center for Complementary and Alternative Medicine

NCCAM (initially the Office of Alternative Medicine) was formed in 1992 by Congress in response to RAND's analysis of spinal manipulation.[31] The mission of NCCAM as stated on its Web site is as follows:

> Explore complementary and alternative healing practices in the context of rigorous science.
>
> Train complementary and alternative medicine researchers.
>
> Disseminate authoritative information to the public and professionals.
>
> NCCAM sponsors and conducts research using scientific methods and advanced technologies to study CAM. CAM is a group of diverse medical and health care systems, practices, and products that are not presently considered to be part of conventional medicine.[33]

World Health Organization

The WFC was accepted for membership in the World Health Organization (WHO) in 1997. A positive recommendation by the World Federation of Public Health Associations (WFPHA) was a large part of the successful application by the WFC.[34] In that recommendation letter, the contribution of chiropractic leaders working within the American Public Health Association (APHA) structure and forming the Chiropractic Health Care section of APHA was cited as an example of how modern chiropractic contributes to the health-care system.[35]

WHO is the United Nations (UN) agency responsible for directing and coordinating international work related to health. It was established in 1948 and has its headquarters in Geneva, Switzerland. Its annual meeting, called the World Health Assembly, is held in Geneva at the UN Palais des Nations each May. WHO is widely regarded as the most successful body in the UN system.

As the WFC explains on its Web site, the relationship between the WFC and WHO is as follows.

Nongovernmental Organizations (NGOs) "These provide many of the human, technical, and financial resources that the WHO relies upon for its work. At present, there are approximately 180 NGOs in official relations with WHO, including charitable organizations (e.g., Aga Khan Foundation, OXFAM, Rotary International, Save the Children Fund, World Vision International) and international organizations representing stakeholders in health care (e.g., International Council of Nurses, International Federation of Pharmaceutical Manufacturers' Associations, the WFC, and the WFPHA). When WFC representatives commenced contacts with WHO in Geneva in 1988, they found that WHO had no knowledge of the chiropractic profession or its growing recognition and contribution to health throughout the world. This was significant for several reasons, including the fact that most governments and their Ministries of Health turn to WHO for advice on matters of legislation relating to health professions. In addition, WHO was sponsoring international meetings in areas of importance to the chiropractic profession without any chiropractic representation such as health human resources or manpower planning and the management of patients with occupational low back pain. Additionally, the chiropractic profession was doing nothing to support the important goals and activities of WHO.

In the years since 1988 that has changed, and collaborative work between the WFC and WHO has included a cosponsored interdisciplinary symposia on Low-Back Pain (London, 1993), The Cervical Spine (Tokyo, 1997), and Chiropractic Education (Philippines, 1998). The WFC has provided various technical papers to WHO, such as "Legislative Approaches to the Regulation of the Chiropractic Profession" (to the WHO Office of Health Legislation) and "The Chiropractic Profession: Principles, Education, Research and Regulation."[34]

APHA

Another positive movement for the profession that came in 1995 was the development of a chiropractic section in the APHA, and its importance is described on the APHA Web site as follows: "APHA is the oldest, largest, and most influential public health association in the United States—and in the world."[35] APHA has been the vehicle by which our profession achieved a much greater level of integration into mainstream health care in the United States. At one time, we had no "seat at the table,"[35] and in fact up until 1983 chiropractic was labeled by APHA as an "unscientific hazard to the health of American citizens,"[35] and an anti-chiropractic policy was widely disseminated to leaders in government and health and to consumer groups. However, thanks to the efforts of the chiropractic leaders within APHA, since 1983 the association has officially recognized chiropractic as "safe and effective for neuro-musculo-skeletal conditions and particularly for low back disorders."[35] Our input is now sought, and we participate in a variety of healthcare programs and projects at the local community, state, national, and international levels thanks to our recognized expertise and status through APHA. Where we were once excluded, we are now invited and welcomed. Chiropractic has had a major impact within APHA, and our active participation has had a major impact on how chiropractic is perceived in the United States and around the world. In fact, our work in APHA is an important part of the history of the chiropractic profession. We will continue to have impact through and within APHA into the future.[35]

Medical Acceptance

In 1998, the *Archives of Internal Medicine* (an American Medical Association [AMA] publication) published an article outlining chiropractic. The authors were not chiropractors; however, the article is illustrative of the optimism conveyed for the chiropractic industry at that time. The authors state the following observation:

> From the first encounter on, chiropractors generate different expectations from conventional physicians. Because conventional practitioners assume that back pain, in the absence of systemic signs, is likely to be self-limited, it is not unusual for a patient to wait weeks for an appointment with a specialist or for radiographic diagnostic assessment. Because a chiropractor believes that back pain is both explicable and amenable to treatment, a patient can usually obtain an appointment within 24 hours of a telephone call. The message of empathy, urgency, comprehension, and support conveyed by such a rapid response is reassuring and provides a heightened sense of care and compassion.[36]

The authors then conclude: "Chiropractic has endured, grown, and thrived in the United States, despite internal contentiousness and external opposition.

Its persistence suggests it will continue to endure as an important component of health care in the United States."

The Wilks Case

The *Wilks* case is familiar to most of those in the chiropractic profession and is a legal battle in which the chiropractic industry filed a formal suit against the AMA that lasted from 1976 to 1987. AMA policy now states that it is ethical for physicians not only to associate professionally with chiropractors but also to refer patients to them for diagnostic or therapeutic services.

Department of Defense

Another benefit is in the more recent inclusion in the Department of Defense. In response to the chiropractic advisory committee, it was recommended that the Office of Research and Development develop an appropriate research agenda for chiropractic care. "In April 2005, the Department of Veterans Affairs announced and requested proposals on chiropractic care research specifically addressing issues such as cost-effectiveness, efficacy, and effectiveness compared to other treatments (head-to-head data) and the best subgroups with which an improvement might be accepted. The VA also indicated that by the end of 2005 employment and hiring directly by the VA would be implemented for chiropractors."[37]

This inclusion is monumental. It would be extremely beneficial if military personnel could attend chiropractic school in exchange for service time as can those studying to be medical practitioners. Currently, the Armed Forces Health Professions Scholarship Program (HPSP) is a scholarship for 2 to 4 years offered to students in schools of medicine, osteopathic medicine, dentistry, and optometry. HPSP students receive full tuition, school-related expenses, and a stipend as benefits.[38] It would certainly be one answer to student loans. Although this is not available presently, it does open the doors for a national VA database of spinal manipulative procedures, which could then be utilized for cohort analysis.

On March 25, 2003, Dr. George McClelland testified to the Department of Veterans Affairs Chiropractic Advisory Committee. His full testimony is available on FCER's Web site.[39] Notably he discusses problems with the medical world and cites statistics for unnecessary surgical procedures and the overutilization of pharmaceuticals. He notes that the House Subcommittee on Oversight and Investigations extrapolated these figures to estimate that, on a nationwide basis, there were 2.4 million unnecessary surgeries performed annually resulting in 11,900 deaths at an annual cost of $3.9 billion.[40] Although these figures are taken from data collected in 1976, their importance is underscored with the 1995 figures citing 250,000 lower back surgeries and U.S. hospital cost of $11,000 per patient and the following conclusion: "This would mean that the total number of unnecessary back surgeries each year in the U.S. could approach 44,000, costing as much as $484 million."[41] In the case of overutilization of prescription medication, Dr. McClelland further quotes that "Total spending on prescription drugs doubled from 1995 to 2000 and tripled from 1990 to 2000, constituting one of the main factors driving up health care expenditures overall."[39] Considering the side effects associated with these medications range from nausea to death, this constitutes a serious problem. I discuss these problems in depth in Chapter 11, "Introduction to Competitive Selling."

Council on Chiropractic Guidelines and Practice Parameters

The Council on Chiropractic Guidelines and Practice Parameters (CCGPP) was formed in 1995 at the behest of the Congress of Chiropractic State Associations and with assistance from the ACA, Association of Chiropractic Colleges, Council on Chiropractic Education, Federation of Chiropractic Licensing Boards, Foundation for the Advancement of Chiropractic Sciences, the FCER, the ICA, National Association of Chiropractic Attorneys, and the National Institute for Chiropractic Research to create an equitable chiropractic practice document. CCGPP was delegated to examine all existing guidelines, parameters, protocols, and best practices in the United States and other nations in the construction of this document. The CCGPP is a tremendous resource for evidence-based chiropractic.

Other Positive Advances

Other positive advances in recent years identified by Nelson et al. include:

- First federally funded chiropractic center for excellence at Palmer University by NIH's NCCAM in 1997
- Publication of the *Headache Report* by Duke University in 2002
- $10 million in federal grants
- Chiropractic services in the military
- Public Law 107-135 enacted on January 23, 2003, for Department of Veterans Affairs[5]

The Bad: Breakdown of Medical Acceptance

Another important component of how we have come to be is how we have evolved. Dr. Scott Haldeman provided a very interesting history when he was a keynote speaker at the 2000 International Conference on Spinal Manipulation.

What is perceived as the first collapse of the bridge between chiropractors and medical doctors is described astutely by Dr. Haldeman: "The most widely quoted theory was that one could seek chiropractic care for anything that was wrong and that chiropractic would make it better. It was also widely believed that everybody should be seeing a chiropractor on a regular basis even if they were healthy. This concept led to the situation where chiropractors became outcasts to the medical system."[14]

Restricted Funding

As Dr. Haas notes in "The White Papers" published in the *Journal of Manipulative and Physiological Therapeutics,* there is currently only one large federally funded research center with both clinical and basic science facilities (Palmer Center for Chiropractic Research) and federal funding remains limited.[7]

Slowed Professional Growth

Nelson et al. state that it was projected that there would be more than 100,000 chiropractors in the United States by 2010.[5] As it happens, the attendance at chiropractic colleges has fallen; although reports that it is again growing have been circulated, we are not on track to grow the profession to 100,000. In fact, at just 66,000 in 2005 we are well short of that goal, especially looking at the numbers of chiropractic graduates being produced each year. In addition, a profession that once enjoyed chiropractic professionals as recruiters for the field has now also diminished. Many students have no family or personal experience with chiropractic. Looming student loans and diminishing fees in a complicated managed care regime continue to scare away many recruits both in allopathic and chiropractic schools.[12]

Chiropractors in Jail

It isn't just the evolution of chiropractic that is of historical interest but also the stand by early chiropractors that is also quite fascinating. An AMA publication reports of less friendlier times for chiropractors.[36]

The authors write of early chiropractic predecessors who in trying to license chiropractic were placed in jail for 90 days charged with "practicing medicine without a license." As the authors note, at the height of the controversy 450 chiropractors were jailed annually. It was the public sympathy spurred by obvious medical entrapment by the medical professionals that saved the plight of early chiropractors. In 1922, there was an overwhelming vote in favor to license chiropractic that resulted in pardoning all chiropractors still in jail. Each state went on fighting for the licensing rights for chiropractors to practice chiropractic. It wasn't until 1970 that federal recognition consolidated state acceptance and conveyed the right to be covered under Medicaid, Medicare, and workers' compensation and granted federal funding for research.

Failed State-Supported Chiropractic College

Another recent blow and wake-up call to the profession came with the cancellation of what was supposed to be the first state-supported chiropractic college at a public university. This could have opened up new opportunities for research, enhanced our cultural authority, opened the doors for a more diverse range of students, and set the precedent for future state-supported colleges.[12] A state-supported college is more affordable to attend than a private college, for tuition, housing, and availability of grants. State-supported colleges would obviously be a major factor in decreasing the student loan burden.

Identity

Despite advancements that have legitimized our profession, we have failed to identify with the identity the public and managed care have given to us and thus in our own internal confusion and differences are now beginning to alienate healthcare professionals. We can't have it both ways: We can't cling to the vitalistic theories of the olden days that lack the research to support them and at the same time state that we are primary care providers. We cannot strive to be included on healthcare plans and then ignore the demands for evidence. We cannot strive to produce evidence on manipulation and be outraged when it isn't in our favor. Health care is not in place for our own personal desires. We have an obligation to continue to learn, to adjust, and to adapt to new evidence, to pull from our clinical experience with the goal being to provide the best care for our patients, whether that calls for manipulation or not.

Evidence-Based Health Care

Chiropractic's future role will probably be determined by its commitment to interdisciplinary cooperation and science-based practice.
—Dr. William Meeker and Dr. Scott Haldeman, *Chiropractic: A Profession at the Crossroads of Mainstream and Alternative Medicine*

The observations of our colleagues and thought leaders in the industry are all saying the same thing: If we don't want to undo all the progress that we have made, we must embrace EBHC and forge relationships with other health disciplines. Some key examples are provided.

As the authors of *Chiropractic as spine care: a model for the profession* states:

> One of the best definitions we have seen appeared in an editorial in the *British Medical Journal* in 1996 written by some of the most prominent educators in EBHC. They defined EBHC as the conscientious, explicit and judicious use of current best external scientific evidence in making decisions about the care of patients.[5, 42]
>
> EBHC principles state that healthcare providers need to combine their clinical expertise with the best available external evidence and that neither alone is sufficient. EBHC stresses the importance of outcomes-based clinical research, of regularly consulting the scientific literature, of optimizing the clinical skills of healthcare providers, and taking patients preferences into account.[5]

As the publication *The Future of Chiropractic Revisited: 2005* points out:

> "Evidence-based and outcomes based medicine is slowly transforming healthcare." All healthcare providers will be fighting for a smaller share. Providers will have to have more than high patient satisfaction rates; they will also have to prove that they are efficacious and cost effective.[12]

Two premier chiropractic institutions for research are the FCER and the Palmer Consortium for Chiropractic Research. To aid the practicing chiropractor, college faculty, researchers, and associations, the FCER is creating the Evidence-Based Chiropractic Resource Center (EB-CRC) to provide education, training, and ready access to information in evidence-based chiropractic care. Components of the virtual EB-CRC include the following:

- A Research Information Center with a digitized, searchable, global database to serve as a resource to the chiropractic community
- Intellectual Property Management Policies and Program, including policies related to recognition rights, publishing, copywriting, and licensing
- Chiropractic College/Program Incubation Services to assist in the development of grant writing, research and trial design, data reduction and analysis, report writing, capital fund raising, and university collaborations with education and research programs and organizations
- Chiropractic College/Program Faculty Training to assist in providing for research education, project and position funding for professionals, career development, and mentoring of student projects
- A Chiropractic Clinical Training Program to provide doctors of chiropractic with education and training (information resources, products, and computer competencies) necessary to practice evidence-based care

- The Chiropractic Professional Association Program to provide information, services, and skills to professional associations to assist in the development of evidence-based programs[43]

Dr. Haas notes in "The White Papers" that political action has been fruitful, resulting in the ongoing funding of HRSA's Chiropractic Demonstration Project, as well as funding for studies of care for the Department of Defense and VA. By law, HRSA requires a chiropractor to serve on its advisory committee, and there has been enhanced funding opportunities from the NCCAM at the NIH.

Why Should You Promote to Medical Physicians?

According to a national survey,[12] back pain is the most prevalent chronic medical problem and accounts for an estimated $50 billion to $100 billion in annual US healthcare costs. With the baby boomer population aging, this problem can be expected to escalate. The competition for treating this group of patients will be extremely competitive, and our role in it is currently being defined and is far from certain.[12] If competition for market share isn't affecting you currently, take the following into consideration. The Institutes of Alternative Futures estimates that in 2002 there were 61,000 chiropractors. The latest trend in chiropractic is 15% growth, meaning that the most current prediction of the population of our workforce is that it will be 70,000 in 2012 (a far cry from earlier industry trends of 100,000 by 2010). Compare this to physical therapists and there is a tremendous trend favoring the growth of physical therapy, not chiropractic. In 2002, there were 137,000 physical therapists, but current trends estimate a 35% increase in that workforce, meaning that by 2012 it is estimated there will be 185,000 physical therapists competing for back pain patients; in plainer terms, chiropractors will be outnumbered 2 to 1. Add to this a projected 77% increase in number of acupuncturists and a 27% increase in the number of massage therapists all fighting for a piece of the pie.

Combine this with the American Physical Therapy Association's (APTA) Vision 2020 goals: "By 2020, physical therapy will be provided by physical therapists who are doctors of physical therapy, recognized by consumers and other health care professionals as practitioners of choice to whom consumers have direct access for the diagnosis of, interventions for, and prevention of impairments, functional limitations, and disabilities related to movement, function, and health."[12, 44] The APTA isn't limiting itself; it is also involved in legislation for direct access, especially for geriatric patients.

The Medicare Patient Access to Physical Therapists Act (HR 1552/S. 932) would improve access to physical therapist services for beneficiaries by eliminating burdensome requirements, such as a physician's referral or certification of the plan of care, as permitted by state law. Currently, 48 states allow physical therapists to evaluate patients without a prior physician's referral, and 43 states and the District of Columbia improve accessibility further by allowing physical therapists to evaluate and treat, under certain conditions, patients without a referral from a physician.[44]

The bottom line of why you should promote is simple: You deserve to have more of the market and you deserve to bring in higher wages. Consumers demand less invasive and more cost-effective health care, and medical doctors want to learn more about our profession. Without a share of voice in the marketplace, our competitors will promote the chiropractor's trade tool and be rewarded with the benefits. The advances in our profession have provided the best sales tools in the form of evidence-based chiropractic. This book will show you how to use them.

REFERENCES

1. Antman EM, Bennett JS, Daugherty A, Furberg C, Roberts H, Taubert KA. Use of nonsteroidal anti-inflammatory drugs. An update for clinicians. A scientific statement from the American Heart Association. *Circulation.* 2007;115:1634–1642. Available at http://circ.ahajournals.org/cgi/content/full/115/12/1634. Accessed December 21, 2007.

2. US Department of Health and Human Services. Defaulted borrowers: Health Education Assistance Loans (HEAL). Available at http://www.defaulteddocs.dhhs.gov/discipline.asp

3. www.PayScale.com

4. Foundation for Chiropractic Education and Research. FCER Funds on Maintenance Care. March 16, 2007. New Release. Available at http://www.FCER.org/html/News/grant0307.htm

5. Nelson CF, Lawrence DJ, Triano JJ, et al. Chiropractic as spine care: a model for the profession. *Chiropractic & Osteopathy.* 2005;13:9.

6. Segall L. Special report: our 9th annual salary and expense survey. *Chiropractic Economics.* 2006;52(6):19. Available at http://www.chiroeco.com/article/2006/Issue6/9thSalarySurvey.pdf. Accessed December 21, 2007.

7. Haas M, Bronfort G, Evans R. The 2006 Chiropractic white papers chiropractic clinical research: progress and recommendations. *J Manipulative Physiol Ther.* 2006; 29:695–706.

8. Bram B. Chiropractic care in California. San Francisco, CA: The Center for the Health Professions, University of California, San Francisco; 2003.

9. Agency for Health Care Policy and Research. Chiropractic in the United States: training, practice and research. Silver Spring, MD: AHCPR; September 1997.

10. Brussee WJ, Willem DC, Assendelft JJ, Breen AC. Communication between general practitioners and chiropractors. *J Manipulative Physiol Ther.* January 2001;24(1):12–16.

11. Shekelle PG, Adams AH, Chassin MR. Spinal manipulation for low-back pain. *Annals of Internal Medicine.* 1992;117(7):590–598.

12. Institute for Alternative Futures. The future of chiropractic revisited: 2005 to 2015. January 2005. Available at http://www.altfutures.com/pubs/Future%20of%20 Chiropractic%20Revisited%20v1.pdf. Accessed December 21, 2007.

13. Quinn J, Lomoriello G. Consumers Union. Which Alternative Treatments Work? 2005. Available at www.chiro.org/alt_med_abstracts/ABSTRACTS/Consumer_Reports_Survey_ shtml

14. American Specialty Health. About us. Available at http://www.ashcompanies.com/ aboutus/. Accessed December 21, 2007.

15. Haldeman S. The Evolution of Chiropractic—Science and Theory. Excerpt from keynote presentation, September 21, 2000. 2000 International Conference on Spinal Manipulation. Reprinted from *FCER Advance,* Winter 2001. Available at www. fcer.org/html/research/Info/haldeman.htm

16. World Federation of Chiropractic. Home page. Available at http://www.wfc.org. Accessed January 2, 2008.

17. Turchin C. Primary care providers: the chiropractic illusion. *Dynamic Chiropractor.* 1994;12(13). Available at http://www.chiroweb.com/archives/12/13/05.html. Accessed January 2, 2008.

18. US Government Accounting Office. Health care access: innovative programs using non-physicians. Report to the Chairman, Special Committee on Aging, US Senate. August 1993.

19. Gaumer G, Walker A, Su S. Chiropractic and a new taxonomy of primary care activities. *J Manipulative Physiol Ther.* 2001;24:239–259.

20. National Board of Chiropractic Examiners. Overview—job analysis of chiropractic 2005. Available at http://www.nbce.org/publications/pub_analysis.html. Accessed December 21, 2007.

21. www.escapehomes.com/main.aspx?tabid=45&temid=186. Baby Boomer Statistics on Empty Nests and Retirement by Del Webb Corp.

22. Soldo BJ, Mitchell OS, Tfaily R, McCabe JF. Cross-cohort differences in health on the verge of retirement. NBER Working Paper No. 12762. December 2006. Available at http://www.nber.org/papers/w12762. Accessed January 2, 2008.

23. http://bhpr.hrsa.gov/interdisciplinary/05chiro.htm. FY2005 Chiropractic Demonstration Projects Program: Elderly Back Pain: Comparing Chiropractic to Medical Care. William Meeker, DC. MPH.

24. National Institutes of Health, National Institute on Aging (NIA). National Institutes of Health. Could Baby Boomers Be Approaching Retirement in Worse Shape Than Their Predecessors? March 5, 2007. Available at www.nih.gov/news/pr/mar2007/nia-05.htm

25. McGinn D, Murr A. Real estate: Not your father's retirement. *Newsweek.* Oct. 23, 2006. Available at www.newsweek.com/ID/72452

26. Schers H, Wensing M, Huijsmans Z, van Tulder M, Grol R. Implementation barriers for general practice guidelines on low back pain. A qualitative study. *Spine.* 2001;26:E348–353.

27. Feise RJ. The path of professionalism. 2002. Available at http://www.chiroevidence.com/Path%20of%20Professionalism.pdf. Accessed January 2, 2008.

28. Langworthy JM, Birkelid J. General practice and chiropractic in Norway: how well do they communicate and what do GPs want to know? *J Manipulative Physiol Ther.* 2001;24:576–581.

29. Mootz R. Chiropractic's current state: impacts for the future. *J Manipulative Physiol Ther.* 2007;30:1–3.

30. Rosner AL. Director of Research testifies at National Institute of Medicine hearings. Foundation for Chiropractic Education and Research. February 27, 2003. Available at http://www.fcer.org/html/Research/IOMtestimony.htm. Accessed January 2, 2008.

31. RAND Health Research Highlights. Changing Views of Chiropractic . . . and a National Reappraisal of Nontraditional Healthcare. 2001. RAND. Available at www.rand.org/pubs/research_briefs/RB4539/index1.html. Accessed January 2, 2008.

32. American Back Society. Home page. Available at http://www.americanbacksoc.org/2006prog.html. Accessed January 2, 2008.

33. National Center for Complementary and Alternative Medicine. NCCAM facts-at-a-glance and mission. Available at http://nccam.nih.gov/about/ataglance/. Accessed January 2, 2008.

34. www.wfc.org/website/WFC/website.nsf/webpage/world_health?opendocument

35. American Public Health Association. Home page. Available at http://www.apha.org/. Accessed January 3, 2008.

36. Kaptchuk T. Chiropractic origins, controversies, and contributions. *Arch Intern Med.* 1998;158:2215–2224.

37. Program Announcement, Request for Applications on Chiropractic Care Research, Department of Veterans Affairs, April 2005. Available at www.research.va.gov/funding/solicitations/docs/chiroprctic_care.pdf

38. Faqs.org. 6. Paying for medical school. Available at http://www.faqs.org/faqs/medicine/education-faq/part2/section-3.html. Accessed January 3, 2008.

39. Foundation for Chiropractic Education and Research. Testimony to the Department of Veterans Affairs Chiropractic Advisory Committee, George B. McClelland, DC. March 25, 2003. Available at www.fcer.org/html/Research/VAtestimony.htm

40. US Congressional House Subcommittee Oversight Investigation. *Cost and Quality of Health Care: Unnecessary Surgery.* Washington, DC: Government Printing Office; 1976.

41. Herman R. Back surgery. *Washington Post.* April 18, 1995:Health section.

42. Sackett DL, Rosenberg WM, Gray JA, Haynes RB, Richardson WS. Evidence based medicine: what it is and what it isn't. *Br Med J.* 1996;312:71–72.

43. FCER Evidence-Based Healthcare a Reality: FCER's EB-CRC to Serve Chiropractic Clinicians, Educators and Researchers. *Advance.* Spring 2007; 25(3). Available at www.FCER.org/Download/Advance/advance0307a.pdf

44. www.apta.org/AM/Template.cfm?Section=Vision_20201&Template=/TaggedPage/TaggedPageDisplay.cfm&TPLID=285&ContentID=32061

Preparing and Executing Your Call: The Who, What, and How of Promoting Your Practice to Physicians

Planning and preparation are key components to a successful sales presentation. These include a thorough understanding of the current research for chiropractic care and knowledge of competitors' strengths and weaknesses. This text includes the necessary information; however, research is always evolving, so it is important to use this text but also to keep abreast of the latest research. Web sites to consult for research updates are included in Appendix B.

In reviewing the research presented in this text, you will become familiar with the key promotional features of chiropractic care and the evidence-based research supporting chiropractic management of neuromuscular disorders. To date the research has primarily focused on acute and chronic lower back pain, acute and chronic neck pain, and headaches. These three conditions make up 95% of the conditions for which patients seek chiropractic care. Attempting to sell and promote less-established research risks 95% of the population just to promote for 5% of the population suitable for a referral. Before we can dive into the research from a promotional standpoint, you need to understand the steps of the selling process, which include the following:

1. Who you should promote to
2. What you should bring to a presentation
3. How to get time with the doctor

Step 1. Who You Should Promote To

The following guidelines can be helpful in determining which practices to promote to:

1. A doctor who has a similar, not necessarily exact, insurance arrangement. For instance, if the doctor's office has 40% of the patients covered under Blue Cross/Blue Shield (BC/BS), you should be a provider of BC/BS. If the doctor is a health maintenance organization (HMO) provider, you should be as well. This can easily be uncovered by calling and asking the doctor's front desk personnel what major insurance companies the doctor takes. Insurance companies' Web sites are also a good source to locate doctors in your area who are also listed as providers under an insurance plan but are not always 100% accurate, nor do they tell you how many patients with that coverage the doctor has. Additionally, you could also ascertain this information from the front staff, which will provide you with a conclusive idea of the office's insurance breakdown. We'll discuss this shortly.

   An examination of your own patients and their feedback on doctors will likely yield similar insurance information.

2. Small offices. It will be less intimidating to start promoting to small offices, and it will allow you time to develop your presentation skills.

3. Specific doctor specialties that are likely to be uninterested themselves in treating back pain such as internal medicine, family practitioners, doctors of osteopathy, orthopedic doctors, psychiatrists, rheumatologists, and sports physicians.

   An important note about Doctors of Osteopathy (DOs). At first consideration, DOs may seem like competitors; however, trends indicate that most DOs do not focus on manipulation. This makes them an ideal referral source because they already understand the importance of manipulation and will be more willing to refer for manipulation. Who may first appear as a competitor may be the most likely first candidate to promote chiropractic to.

4. A doctor within a close geographical area.

5. Calling local physical therapy offices that do not also have a chiropractor in the facility and asking them which doctors refer to them can be a way to find out which doctors are likely to refer out.

Step 2. What You Should Bring to a Presentation

After you have identified the doctors you will be contacting, you will want to gather some sales aids. There are several types of sales aids, and the following will be most helpful:

- Detail binder
- Master visual aids (MVAs)
- Clinical reprints
- Prescription pads
- Competitive information
- Managed care information
- Your practice information

Each of these sales aids is discussed in more detail in the following subsections.

Detail Binders

Detail binder is a sales term. When you are communicating material, you are providing details and your binder holds all of the "details" or promotional points of your service. Your detail binder is a collection of supporting materials for several components of your promotional progression and without doubt is mostly composed of many clinical reprints, many of which are discussed in this text. Detail binders change as new information and research become available. In general, the following information should be in your binder and arranged by topic:

- Safety data
- Efficacy data. Include the main papers that you think are strong, such as one or two papers for each of the areas that have been proved efficacious. At this time, that is lower back (acute and chronic), neck (acute and chronic), and headaches.
- Cost-effectiveness data.
- Mechanism of action for manipulation.
- Patient intake forms and examination forms.
- Objective outcome measurements such as the Oswestry Disability Index and Neck Disability Index.
- Description of the chiropractic education. The objective is not to try to prove that the chiropractor's education is equal to or better than the medical doctor's; rather, it should serve to illustrate the well-rounded

and intensive academic curriculum. It isn't necessary to compare the chiropractic curriculum to the medical curriculum.

- Your curriculum vitae. Include your professional associations, personal accomplishments, papers you have published, awards, and so forth.

All of the data in the binder, with the exception of your curriculum vitae and chiropractic education, is covered in depth in the research portion of this book. To gather chiropractic educational information, one should consult your alma mater for the specifics of the curriculum.

Master Visual Aids

An MVA is a snapshot of research material that highlights important points taken from clinical data you think worthy of promoting to the doctor. The MVA is more colorful and the graphs are larger than what you see in the clinical reprint so that important information stands out. An MVA is typically printed on high-gloss sturdy stock paper. An MVA can be homemade, but it should not look homemade. Be mindful of copyright laws if you choose to create your own. Both Aligned Methods and the American Chiropractic Association have MVAs available for purchase. More information is available in Appendix A.

Although an MVA is useful to make a brief presentation impactful, it should not be a replacement for a clinical study. Whether the presentation is from an MVA or a clinical study, the study design and its specifics should still be provided verbally to the doctor. How to do this is discussed later in the text. Whatever clinical is covered in the MVA should be *readily* available as a clinical reprint to leave with the physician or at least it should be available to pull out for a more thorough discussion.

Different personalities react differently to sales aids, and a guide on how to present to different types of personalities is provided in Chapter 4. It can benefit you to have both a detail binder and an MVA with which to make your point. Note the doctors' reaction to both and determine which one seems to draw the doctor in.

It is important that an MVA always cover three major components of manipulation: Safety, efficacy, and cost-effectiveness. Because one MVA may illustrate two separate graphs from two separate studies, it is important not to combine them verbally to come up with one conclusion. Suppose an MVA illustrates two studies in two separate charts with the following findings:

Study 1: A study of manipulation compared to placebo for chronic lower back pain illustrates statistically significant findings in favor of manipulation based on the Oswestry Disability Score, which demonstrated a 60% improvement in scores.

Study 2: A study of acupuncture compared to placebo for chronic lower back pain illustrates statistically significant findings in favor of acupuncture based on the Oswestry Disability Score, which demonstrated a 30% improvement in scores.

Would it be okay, based on these findings, to say that manipulation is better than acupuncture for chronic lower back pain because it provided more improvement in the Oswestry Disability Scores? If your answer is yes, you need to rethink your strategy. A doctor will not buy into this conclusion and will most likely tell you that you can't compare apples to oranges. By this, the doctor means that the study populations are different, the administration of care might have been different, and the outcome was pooled differently.

Meta-analysis, pooled studies, and true head-to-head studies are appropriate types of studies to use to compare the efficacy of one treatment to another. Chapter 8 discusses which clinical studies are available to compare manipulation directly to another treatment.

In summary, an MVA provides the media format that allows you to cover multiple selling features from multiple sources in one convenient location.

Clinical Reprints

Clinical reprints are your primary promotional tool. They are useful to leave with a clinician as a reminder of your conversation, to help you recall and reference information that supports a study, or to leave for a physician that you simply can't access. Clinical reprints should not be photocopies and they should be free of any markings because if you hand over a study in which you have highlighted certain areas, it could be presumed that you are focusing only on the positive findings and attempting to divert attention away from the negative findings. It is okay if there is negative information in the study; in a way it makes the study more legitimate because it demonstrates the authors recognize both the strengths and the weaknesses. Reprint order information is always listed near the beginning or end of a study, and many journal Web sites include information on how to order reprints.

Prescription Pads

You will want to provide the doctor with prescription pads that include information about your office. The prescription pads should list your hours and days of operations and directions to your office. You can bring several pads so that you have enough for the doctor to make one available in each treatment room as well as at the nurses' station. You should allow an area for comments and provide a list of treatment areas with a box for check marking. A sample copy is available in Appendix I. You may feel compelled to provide the doctor with thick tablets, and in fact this may make them more noticeable. I suggest you might provide the doctor with a tablet of 25 sheets or so. It makes for a good excuse to show up at the office and talk with the doctor if you are there for the purpose of replenishing stock. If you have established good rapport and referrals are coming in, go with the thicker pads. Both are suitable; just make sure you provide them. Don't be surprised if despite this tool doctors just write orders on their own personal prescription pads.

Competitive Information

This is not meant to be confused with competitive information that you would find in a clinical. Instead, this means you examine your local competition and have some competitive data available. For instance, when you talk with the front desk person (more on this soon), you may uncover that the office primarily refers to XYZ Physical Therapy. You should call XYZ Physical Therapy or visit it. You can then ask them the following questions:

- What insurance do you take, including workers' compensation and personal injury?
- What is your first available treatment?
- What services do you offer?
- What is the background of the therapist who is providing the care?
- Do you require preauthorizations and do you do them on behalf of the doctor's office?

Knowing this type of specific competitive information provides a promotional selling feature for your office. For instance, you may be willing to do any necessary preauthorizations. You will most likely be able to see a patient sooner than the physical therapist can. These are all features that "beat" the competition without bashing the competition.

It would also be helpful to compare the chiropractic and physical therapy insurance benefits that this doctor is most concerned about. This includes preauthorization requirements, maximum number of office visits, and out-of-pocket expenses. You may find that a certain insurance company provides better coverage for chiropractic care, more annual benefits, or no preauthorization requirements, which can delay when the patient can first be seen for care.

Another example of competitive information might be medication related. If you uncover through the front desk that this doctor often prescribes cyclobenzaprine, you should be prepared to know the side effects, cost, and drug-to-drug profile associated with it.

Having a copy of the medications product insert (available on Web sites such as Drugstore.com) or writing up the standard wait times for a local physical therapy office or any other key features that distinguish your office serve as a visual aid. These aids should note the date that the information was current.

Managed Care Information

As you begin to familiarize yourself with a certain doctor's office you will want to determine the specifics about managed care. It makes no sense to pick a doctor who is heavily involved in HMO contracts if you are not. In addition, closely matching your own managed care information in your sales detail makes your data more applicable to the doctor's patients. You can print out a sheet that covers all of the insurance types that you take or have billed for. List them in as much detail as possible. If the doctor asks what, for example, a Blue Cross/Blue Shield patient will pay for care at your office, you can locate BC/BS in your data and quote the possible deductible and co-pay ranges as well as any annual visit caps. If you don't have the information, or if it takes up too much room, make sure you return at a later time and give the doctor the information. Again, your office information can be compared to other available treatment options such as physical therapy coverage. It isn't necessary to match the doctors' insurance plans 100%, but just make sure you match the big ones.

This brings up a potential selling point if the benefits are the same for, say, physical therapy and chiropractic. For example, how would you handle a doctor if he or she said to you:

> "The financial data are the same for PT and chiropractic care. My patients have done well with PT, so I don't know why I would switch and send them to you."

The answer is the efficacy of manipulation. This type of question opens the door to presenting the data on efficacy, especially data that directly compare physical therapy and chiropractic manipulation.

It is certainly a good rapport builder and selling advantage if you are willing to take the burden of preauthorizations and insurance calls off of the doctor's staff's plate. In most cases, preauthorizations are not necessary for chiropractic care, and this is an advantage of chiropractic care over any care that requires preauthorizations, such as physical therapy. Once you verify insurance, you will then be able to contact the patient to schedule care, making it very convenient for the patient. Make sure your staff understands that the faster you turn this around, the more impressive it is to the doctor and his or her patients.

One final note on managed care: You need to illustrate that you treat and release your patients. Guidelines are available for chiropractors on reasonable treatment plans such as a moderate lower back sprain. You can likewise provide the doctor with some rough guidelines on treatment for common chiropractic problems and allow this to cross over into information on potential costs for a particular insurance patient.

Do not promote maintenance care. Not only does the chiropractic profession lack research data supporting maintenance care, but we have long-term study data on back pain that show patients had lower recurrence rates with manipulation without having maintenance care. You can't sell efficacy and promote the fact that chiropractic patients enjoyed longer periods of relief even after they completed treatment and then turn around and promote maintenance care.

In the event a patient has no chiropractic coverage, many chiropractors feel sympathy for the patient and want to offer cash discounts. A word of caution: Please check with your state licensing board and the American Chiropractic Association before proceeding with any offerings of cash discounts. There are many situations in which it is illegal, unethical, or a potential cause for losing a preferred provider status with an insurance company.

Your Practice Information

Include your hours, major insurance contracts, staff names, and office location. This information may also include where you refer for special imaging. Providing your direct line and emergency information is helpful so that if the doctor needs you, he or she has a direct and personal link to you. Keep your practice information in your binder and also available as a handout.

This practice information is for the doctor, not the patient. The prescription pads are for the patient, and any further information on your services for patients can be provided directly by your office staff.

Step 3. How to Get Time with the Doctor

There will be a time as you start this process that you pause to take a deep and nervous breath. It occurs the minute you prepare to open the door to the doctor's office for the first time. Although it can be unnerving to step out of your comfort level, these moments are fleeting. Remember, the worst that can happen is the doctor says "no." If that happens, reevaluate what might have gone wrong. You may have the opportunity to fix it with the same doctor, or you may decide to move on to another office. Let's take a look at what happens once you push through the office door for the first time.

Getting Past the Gatekeepers

The front desk personnel at physicians' offices truly are the gatekeepers, and they can be tough to get past. Many times the front desk staff are ignored, pestered, yelled at, or worse. Because you are a doctor, you may assume that they will be friendlier to you, but this isn't always true.

Once you walk into the office, introduce yourself to the front desk personnel as "Dr. _____" so that you can establish some authority and respect. I have observed other medical doctors introduce themselves this way, so it isn't out of the ordinary. You can also present a business card to them. An appropriate and standard first contact example follows:

> "My name is Dr. Acampora. I was wondering if I could slip back into the halls and introduce myself to Dr. _____?"

If they welcome you in, don't just step back to meet the doctor but first gather some facts from the front desk. Ask them politely for this information:

- What insurance do they take? (Hopefully, you have called ahead to ascertain whether this office is a good fit for your purposes as discussed earlier.)
- What are their hours? (If when you meet the doctor and he asks for you to come after hours, you will already have a time in mind and you will know if it works in your schedule; additionally, you might identify a similar time that you each have open.)
- What local orthopedist and neurologist do they refer to?
- What physical therapy practice do they utilize for their patients?
- Who does their insurance preauthorizations? (Try to meet this person first to see what types of problems he or she has with medicine and physical therapy authorizations such as length of time for preauthorizations or more than a day for a first visit.)
- What local chiropractor or acupuncture doctor do they refer to? (This should give you some instant feedback!)
- Do they see a lot of back pain patients?
- Do they bill for workers' compensation?

Obviously, you don't want to just fire question after question at them, but you also want to get some competitive information and some points that may serve as selling features for your presentation if the doctor happens to have time to talk with you right away.

Lunches and Dinners

It is not necessary to purchase lunch or dinner for the doctor, especially if you are on a limited budget. You can set up an appointment to meet with the doctor one on one at a time that works for both of you. The entire purpose of this book is to offer chiropractic professionals a cost-effective tool that allows you to build your practice. According to the National Board of Chiropractic Examiners 2005 Job Analysis, chiropractors spend roughly $1,000 a month on advertising.[1] A portion of this money could make a more direct hit if it was spent on lunches or dinner engagements to help develop rapport and relationships with medical professionals. Spending $50 on lunch with a doctor in a small office who has patients to refer seems like a better choice than spending $500 on a direct mail flyer. This is an optional approach, but for offices that you are having difficulty getting past the gatekeeper or getting time with the doctor, bringing lunch to them may get you in the front door.

If you decide to make a lunch meeting, the following can guide you through the specifics of setting up a lunch appointment. At the front desk, you can say the following:

> "I would like to bring in lunch to the office. Who can I talk to so that I may set this up?"

This may sound presumptive, but there are very few doctors' offices that refuse a free lunch. Doctors and their office staff have limited time to go out and get lunch for themselves, so this is usually well received by the office staff. Once you are in front of the person who schedules lunches, ask when the next available lunch is. The person will reply in one of the following ways:

- The doctor has to first okay the lunch.
- We don't do lunches.
- Our lunches are booked a year in advance. (Busy or popular offices open their lunch schedule October through December to book all lunches for the following year.)
- We have one available in 2 weeks.

If the office does not do lunches, smile nicely and say:

> "I understand. Perhaps I can offer to take the doctor out to dinner. What is one of the doctor's favorite restaurants?"

(For more information on ethics, refer to Chapter 3.)

If their lunches are booked well in advance, ask to be put down to cover a lunch that cancels at the last minute, or find out if they might make an exception to allow you to bring breakfast. Find out if the doctor goes out to dinner with colleagues, and then find out one of the doctor's favorite spots. It might be an opportunity to take the doctor and a couple of the doctor's colleagues out to dinner and talk to all of them about chiropractic care. Typically, in a dinner situation you discuss the challenges verbally and present information verbally. It is not well received to pull out a detail binder at a restaurant and present data. Of course, as the meal ends, ask the doctor or doctors if you could meet with them individually at their office to share the evidence with them.

Don't assume that an existing pharma lunch prohibits you from talking with the doctor during the meal. Many times as a rep I invited the doctor's colleague to lunch too and presented to both of them because I knew it would allow me more time with my primary target. You could be that other doctor. More important, just because a rep brought lunch does not imply that he or she will monopolize the doctor's entire lunch hour. Some doctors give the rep 5 minutes while they fill up their plate (usually a larger office), while others sit and eat with them (usually in an office with no more than two doctors). Even if the doctor sits down to eat, the lunch will likely be over in a half hour, so there is still time to talk to you.

The difference between a successful lunch or dinner and an unsuccessful one is whether you commanded the time you deserved. Did you just provide a free and fun lunch, or did you actually provide information? Providing information is imperative for the doctor and provides a service. Otherwise, you're just a nice person, and it might be a while before you get more time with the doctor. If you provided something of value, then the doctor is more likely to value your visits.

If you do book a lunch, indicate to the front desk that you will call a few days in advance to find out what people might like to have. The following information is important:

- Are there any food allergies?
- Are there any dietary restrictions, or is anyone a vegetarian?
- How many people are in the office?
- What time should the food arrive? What time will the doctor break for lunch?
- What are some caterers or lunch spots that they are fond of?

The reason you should call in advance is that many of these offices have lunch meetings every day and chain-store sandwiches may be greeted with little enthusiasm if that is what they have had all week. Calling ahead to see what they have had will help your lunch be greeted with enthusiasm and is a thoughtful thing to do. You can contact local caterers to ask if they do "pharm rep lunches." The caterer will understand that there are financial budgets to work with and they are familiar with setting up in doctors' offices. Catering a lunch is not as expensive as you might think, and it certainly does not have to be extravagant. Catering is much preferred to spending your own time picking up lunch and bringing it in, which requires you also provide drinks, flatware, and plates.

The front desk personnel may mention that they also do breakfast appointments, which can work exactly like lunches do. Overall, I have not found providing breakfast to be a good return on the dollar. Doctors may have just completed rounds at the hospital or may be late returning from the hospital and already have patients loaded up in the treatment rooms. Their mind is ready to start treating patients and not necessarily ready to learn information. The time they give you may be significantly less, but if that is the only time you can get, take it.

Meeting the Doctor

When you enter the back hallways, there is typically a nurse's station. For a small practice, this may be a filing cabinet in the middle of the hallway. Introduce yourself as a doctor to a nurse or staff member so that they understand you aren't a sales representative, and tell them you are there to quickly introduce yourself to the physician. Ask them where the best place for you to stand is. If a doctor emerges and is still discussing patient care with the patient, you should discreetly turn your back or move away to honor the patient's privacy. The same should be done if you are standing near the scale and a nurse needs to weigh a patient. When the doctor steps out, attempt to make eye contact with the doctor to politely get his or her attention. Don't be surprised if the doctor tries to ignore you; they probably think you are a rep. Eventually, doctors know they need to greet you. Greet the doctor with appropriate enthusiasm and get right to the point. You can use the following as a first attempt:

> "Hello, Dr. _____. My name is _____ and I am a chiropractor located on Everett Road. I wanted to stop by and introduce myself and my services. As you know, many patients are interested in alternative care and recent warnings on medications are fueling that interest. Are you familiar with any of the evidence-based research on manipulation?"

Pause to see how the doctor responds. Either the doctor will be very positive or at worst will say he or she is really not interested or gruffly tells you he or she doesn't like chiropractors.

If the response is positive, indicate that you have or can make a lunch appointment, or ask the doctor if he or she would prefer to go out to dinner. If the response is really positive, the doctor might give you 10 minutes right away. Be sure you have come prepared with your detail binder and clinicals.

If the response is negative, try the following approach:

> "I understand, in the past, there have been substantial discon-
> nects between our two professions. With the trend for health care
> now focused on evidence-based health care, I thought I might try
> to bridge this gap by sharing the evidence on manipulation for the
> conditions for which it has proven to be effective. Would you
> share some of your insight on chiropractic with me? I would like
> to try to understand your position."

This should be delivered in a voice that is not adversarial and that inflects genuine concern and interest in the doctor's position.

This approach would be very hard for a doctor to walk away from. In a way, you have been blessed with an objection right out of the gate and it gives you an opportunity right there to try to turn the call around. Empathy and sympathizing are your best defense. If you try to understand why the doctor feels that way, you can reference the information in your detail binder that you have to overcome the doctor's objections. Let's assume for the moment that the doctor thinks chiropractors are unsafe. You can make the following points:

> "Doctor, I understand the amount of negative press chiropractors
> have endured from the media highlighting a few cases. I have
> strong evidence from reputable medical journals, such as the
> American Heart Association's publication *Stroke,* that examines
> safety as well as studies printed in *Spine* that examine the effi-
> cacy of manipulation. Do you have 10 minutes to briefly examine
> the findings?"

By sympathizing with the doctor, you have uncovered the reason behind an objection, and by utilizing the evidence you are overcoming the objection with professionalism. It is perfectly acceptable to cover these data if time permits, and if not to express concern that the doctor receives the true evidence on safety and not sensationalism by the media. You need to be careful that you aren't challenging the doctor's perceptions and ask for 10 minutes of time to give the doctor the real facts and evidence on chiropractic. At this point, you are just trying to get a commitment to discuss the evidence. In rare cases, you may just get a doctor who doesn't want to hear your information no matter what you do. In such cases, you may just want to move on to another doctor's office.

Even in a negative encounter make sure you leave a clinical that deals with efficacy and safety along with a note such as the following:

Dear Dr. _____,

It was a pleasure to meet you yesterday, and I am very appreciative that you were honest enough to share your insights on chiropractic and safety with me. I do understand why you have your beliefs on chiropractic, and I am sorry that such disconnect still exists between our two professions. Although you may not send your back pain patients to a chiropractor, they may seek care on their own. If a patient mentions he or she is seeking chiropractic care, I wanted to make sure that you have been provided with the most conclusive safety data on manipulation. Enclosed is a study from *Stroke* in which the authors concluded that "the rarity of VBAs makes this association difficult to study despite high volumes of chiropractic treatment."[2] I hope you will not hesitate to call me in the future if you are interested in learning more about the evidence on manipulation and how it might be a beneficial treatment for your patients.

Respectfully,

_____, DC

If you know that the doctor likes Starbucks coffee, leave the information with a fresh Starbucks coffee if you are so inclined; it may get more attention that way. Provide a study on safety and one on chronic lower back pain or an MVA. Even if doctors look at your information only briefly, something might catch their eye.

For those who want to get medical referrals but who are too intimidated to make an in-person sales pitch, this approach of providing information through a letter with a personalized snack may work well. For as many doctors as you can, make an effort each day to drop off an introductory package to a few physicians with some type of snack or coffee to enjoy while they read the material. You could call the day before and explain to the staff that you will be doing this and find out what time would be good to drop off a coffee or a sandwich. Make sure the snack is something the doctor will like. Then, create a basic promotional package that includes a clinical on lower back pain as well as an MVA that covers the same information in addition to some safety data. In such cases, your introductory letter may read as follows:

Dear Dr. —————,

My name is —————, DC. I am a chiropractor located two blocks away on the corner of Jackson and Everett Roads.

In February 2007, the American Heart Association published safety data on the use of NSAIDs in treating patients who are at risk for or who have heart disease or stroke. The guidelines printed in their journal *Circulation* indicate that NSAIDs should be one of the last treatment option for this patient group. I have included this article for your review.

Manipulation for chronic lower back pain has some compelling and strong evidence. I have included an article from —————— [name the journal article, preferably one on chronic lower back pain because it is presumed to be safe by most MDs and chronic back pain is difficult to treat. Provide a very brief conclusion and leave the clinical reprint of the study. If you have one, an MVA that reiterates the main findings of this same study and that also has safety data would be appropriate as well.]

I would like to extend an offer for lunch in your office or dinner* at a restaurant to share some of the evidence on manipulation and how chiropractic care might benefit your patients that are no longer candidates for long-term NSAID use. Please feel free to contact me to set up a time to meet at your convenience.

Sincerely,

—————, DC

*In this case bring your evidence to dinner because it may be your only opportunity to present it.

A paper presentation is a slower sales process and has less impact. The doctor may have an unwarranted negative presumption of chiropractic care and may never contact you. With a face-to-face sales approach, you immediately uncover objections and overcome them utilizing professionalism and supportive evidence-based research. Again, promotion must be based on your comfort level, and you have two options to begin the process of getting medical referrals. I encourage you to step out of your comfort level because the results will be much faster and you will be more satisfied with the process and subsequent outcome.

The next chapters look at a formal detail with a doctor and reveal a conversational selling model to use as a guide in your sales or promotional efforts. We also look at selling styles and how to change your approach based on personalities. In the research section of this book, an outline of how to present a clinical study and discuss studies that do well in front of physicians is presented.

REFERENCES

1. National Board of Chiropractic Examiners. Job analysis of chiropractic 2005. A project report, survey analysis, and summary of the practice of chiropractic within the United States. January 2005. Available at http://www.nbce.org/publications/pub_analysis.html. Accessed October 13, 2006.

2. Rothwell D, Bondy S, Williams J. Chiropractic manipulation and stroke: A population-based case-control study. *Stroke.* 2001;32:1054–1060.

Chapter 3

Introducing a Conversational Sales Model

W hy will a conversational sales model work? Initiating a two-way dialogue allows the exchange of information and the ability to elicit and
overcome misperceptions and objections from the person to whom
you are selling, which allows your promotional efforts to be heard and understood. Many people are too intimidated to take on any type of a conversational sales approach. For some it conjures up a negative image, but as you
will see in this chapter, it can be done with professionalism and integrity. For
others it conjures the fear of being on the spot to answer tough questions;
however, as you will learn you won't always know the answer and this is okay
as long as you are willing to research the question and provide the answer at
a later date. The sales model between two physicians focuses on an exchange
of educational information and introduces the art and subtleties of checking
in with your audience for their agreement and eventually their commitment.
Medical doctors are very familiar with this process and will readily accept it.
Most forms of sales with physicians—from pharmaceuticals to orthopedics to
marketing to software—typically use a face-to-face encounter. Securing time
with a physician is your best opportunity for success.

The need for chiropractors to promote their services was discussed exten-
sively in Chapter 1. The way in which we can successfully promote our services
is provided in this chapter. In today's healthcare trend of using evidence-based
health care, we let the research speak for itself. Using a conversational sales
model, we can uncover the medical world's objections and from there decide
which research is most applicable for particular physician practices. The
selling process is known as a needs-based sale and focuses on creating a
need for your service or product through open conversation. It is an engaging process that encourages physicians to illustrate their thought process on
how they use referral sources and treatment options for their patients. It is a
process that allows you to exchange information based partly on assumptions

as well as information you gain from the physician during the course of the conversation. As such, you have a customizable protocol that can be altered based on time, personality, and content. The selling process is only as good as your research, and your research is only as good as how you communicate it, and your time to communicate is only as good as its applicability to the physicians and their patients.

Introducing the Needs-Based Sale

There are several components of the needs-based sale and as many ways to present it. The following is a rough guideline—and is provided only as a guideline! In its strictest format it would be robotic and hardly conversational. Once you learn the outline, though, you will soon be able to utilize it as a guide throughout your presentations. Sometimes you may rearrange the steps to fit the conversation, or they may not be appropriate based on the buy-in from the physician. It is a sales call outline, but to the casual observer it is just a conversation and that is how it should feel when you are promoting.

Throughout this text you will find a common theme: The necessity to precall plan. Every doctor is different and your presentation will be based on the physician's specialty, insurance information, competitive information, and practice profile. The result is a variety of approaches aimed at placing chiropractic as a first-line choice. Chapter 2 discusses what you need to bring for your sales call and how to uncover useful information from the front desk personnel. This chapter discusses how to deliver an appropriate sales message and how to confidently change it on the spot as you uncover the objections the doctor may present in a manner the doctor's personality will respond to.

The Goal of the Sales Call

The primary goal of the sales call is to identify which message you want to deliver. The first call should clearly focus on uncovering the physician's needs and educating the physician on the mechanism of manipulation. As you do this, you will uncover information to further your sales call that can include the physician's area of interest (lower back vs. neck), what type of material the physician responds to (clinical paper or master visual aid), how to the deliver the message (in depth or briefly), and what the doctor's perception of chiropractic is (safety issues, efficacy issues, financial issues, or if the doctor simply does not know enough about our profession to utilize it as a treatment option). This may take one or several calls to accomplish based on buy-in, the amount of detail you need to cover, and the time you have to do it in. At first your visits to the physician may be rather frequent. Then once you are established as a reputable choice for referring patients, the visits will start to spread out.

Promotions 101

There are a few basic issues that apply on every promotional call:

1. You should say "manipulation by a chiropractor" as often as possible. For instance, state: "The patients who had manipulation by a chiropractor experienced a 60% improvement in their Oswestry scores" rather than, "The patients had a 60% improvement in their Oswestry scores." Literally, this is like a commercial. The more you say what it is you are promoting, the more it will sink in to the listener. Manipulation is a powerful tool for back pain, so give it due credit. Chiropractors are the most well trained and most experienced in delivering manipulation, so make sure you give yourself due credit. Saying only "manipulation" doesn't emphasize the fact that doctors should send patients to you especially because our competitors use manipulation. When the doctor thinks *manipulation,* the doctor should just as quickly think *chiropractic manipulation.* The exception to this is when manipulation in a study you are presenting was not performed by chiropractors exclusively.

   Likewise you want to downplay and limit your use of competitors' name. I once went into an office where my pharmaceutical sales numbers were slowly growing. The competitor who used to have the lead until my product took over had just left, and the doctor said to me: "Your competitor was just in here talking about your product more than their own product, but I protected you." I doubt this was the case; rather, the competition just said my product's name so much it sounded more like a sell for me than against me. The lesson here is that the doctor recalled my product in the sales call, not the competitor's, and worse for the competitor the doctor started to protect my product and the justification he had for using it first line. In other words, the doctor sold himself on my product. Had the competition mentioned its own product as much as it mentioned mine, it might have had more impact.

2. Always mention a patient type. It adds more impact to utilize a specific patient type: Say "patients in their mid-40s with nonradicular back pain over 6 months" rather than "chronic back pain patients." This is referred to as painting a patient picture. You literally want a patient type or even a specific patient to pop into the mind of the physician. This adds substantial impact because the next time the

doctor sees this type of patient your services will also pop into his or her mind. Any issue in health care always relates back to patients to meet their healthcare needs in an unbiased manner that offers them safe, economical, and effective forms of treatment.

For instance, reverse the selling process to one in which you are being sold to. The salesperson represents disposable muscle stimulation pads and is attempting to get you to switch brands. They can offer you a "commercial" such as the following scenario:

> "Dr. Acampora, XYZ muscle stim pads are the newest and easiest pads to use. They work as well as the ones you use now with no rashes because of an aloe base. Can I leave you with some samples today to get you started?"

Or the salesperson can uncover a problem with your current choice and create a need for you to switch to XYZ muscle stim pads. In the following situation, the sales rep has pre-call planned and knows that the pads you use have a 15% association with skin reactions; the goal is to get you to try the product when your patient experiences a rash, which will prove to be a positive experience.

> Rep: "Dr. Acampora, for patients who need muscle stim, but who also have very sensitive skin, reactions to stim pads must be a problem. What are your other treatment options?"

> I reply: "I would probably switch over to ultrasound."

> Rep: "XYZ muscle stim pads have been shown to be as comfortable for patients and as effective at dispersing treatment as your current choice. However, XYZ pads have an aloe-based adhesive that solves the problem of dermatitis associated with other pads. If resolving the dermatitis allowed you to continue with your first treatment of choice, would you consider trying XYZ muscle stim pads for patients who have a skin reaction with your current choice?"

3. Stop, pause, and listen! This is very important. You literally need to pause after asking questions or delivering important data, especially for doctor types who may need to silently mull over your information. It may feel uncomfortable, but it may also save your call. If you don't allow them to speak or give them time to answer, you are not only providing a commercial but you are preventing any chance of uncovering their thoughts or opinions on the data you are giving them. If you talk over that pause and continue on with a patient type that might not be applicable to their practice, your entire presentation may mean nothing to them.

4. Promote based on the facts. If you don't have the research to support your claim, you simply won't be in a position to promote the service. As doctors, we all have a legal and ethical duty to offer the most current up-to-date care based on clinical experience and research literature. When doctors are open to learning about a new treatment option, they will weigh the risk to benefit ratio of the treatment before prescribing it to their patients. Certainly, we do the same thing when we create treatment plans for our patients. Salesmanship in health care is more of an educational tour of a product, or in our case, a service and procedure. The evidence must be strong and from a reputable source. There is no "spinning" of data here. The "sales" process associated with health care involves uncovering the doctors' needs to see if there are needs that your service can meet for the doctors' patients and promoting the facts on why your service may be a better choice. If you proceed in this manner and you convincingly relate your material to the appropriateness of patient care, you can and will begin the formation of a strong professional relationship.

5. Clarifying questions are your safety harness. When you are met with a question that you don't have an answer for, you need to stop and clarify. This is discussed in detail shortly.

The Conversational Sales Model

Now that you have a goal in mind and some of the sales basics covered, let's take a look at the sales model.

The main steps of any sales process are as follows:

1. Introduction, which consists of information gathering or probing questions to gain an understanding of the doctor's current thoughts and opinions. In addition, the probing questions will provide an idea on what data would be most appropriate to present. For instance:

   - "Dr. XX, thank you for your time today. I was hoping you could tell me what your thoughts or experiences are about chiropractic care."

   - "So that I might understand where chiropractic care would fit into your care regimen, what is your treatment protocol for a chronic lower back pain patient?

   - "Have you seen any data on manipulation, or do you know what the mechanism of action is for manipulation and why it works?"

   Once you have a good idea on what the doctor does know and what you could show him or her to improve on that knowledge, you can continue probing the doctor on what some of his or her treatment challenges are. For instance:

- "Doctor, you mentioned that you refer chronic lower back pain patients to physical therapy. What benefit are you looking for?"
- "Do you find that patients must wait while preauthorizations are acquired, for insurance?"

2. Presentation of data based on the feedback you have obtained. At this point, the process moves from probing questions to feedback questions. For instance, if you present data on chronic lower back pain and you want to find out if the doctor agrees with the baseline outcome measures, you can check in with the doctor by asking him: "Do you see the same type of scores with your own patients?"

3. Closing. In the past, it was recommended that you ask for the doctor's commitment such as, "Doctor, do I have your commitment that you will utilize chiropractic before sending a patient to physical therapy?" This is tacky. Rather, summarize your data, such as, "Dr. XX, the data for chiropractic manipulation illustrated a rapid and robust response to care for chronic lower back pain. You indicated that the baseline scores were similar to what you see with your own patients. I also accept walk-in patients or I can schedule an appointment for your patients within 24 hours, which would solve the long wait times you currently experience." Then close such as, "Based on this information, would you consider chiropractic care for your chronic low back pain patients?" Typically, the doctor will respond, "Yes," or "It looks really good." If he or she starts asking insurance questions or how to refer patients over, then you already have a commitment. If you sense hesitation or lack of buy-in, you can ask the doctor what might prevent him or her from referring a patient. At this point, you might have to get back into another clinical paper and repeat steps 2 and 3.

Opening Statements

Opening statements consist of statements about symptoms that create a perceived need for chiropractic services and plant a seed for change from the physician's current treatment choice to chiropractic manipulation by demonstrating an unmet treatment need by the competition. Typically, the opening statement paints a picture of a specific patient type, which serves to place your service in the doctor's mind when he treats this patient. A seed of doubt is a subtle statement that identifies a weakness or problem with a current therapeutic choice.

The opening statement serves as a transition from an introduction and information gathering to creating the base of your sales message. It should not be vague but specific. Take the following example into consideration.

> "Dr. XX, chiropractic can work on many types of musculoskeletal conditions and it is proven to be safe and effective. How have you been treating musculoskeletal conditions?"

In the preceding example, the doctor is going to have to ask you questions to figure out how to answer your question. It is too vague and the answer could be anything. However, in the following example a specific patient type is identified, allowing you more control of the conversation. In this example, a specific picture of a patient is painted, and the stage is set for a specific competitor and unmet treatment need.

> "Dr., Blue Cross patients presenting with a recurrent bout of lower back pain within 6 months of a previous episode can be difficult to treat. Patients experiencing chronic pain don't want to wait a couple of weeks for a physical therapy appointment, and delay in treatment can lead to a longer duration of pain. Help me understand how you differentiate between treatment strategies for these patients."

Probe/Assumptive Statements

Probes are essentially questions that serve to uncover physicians' reasons and practice philosophy on how they treat a particular problem. Probes help to uncover what physicians like about their first-line treatment choice, their experiences that have created the choice of this treatment, and any problems they run into administering this treatment.

This is the step that gets the sales process flowing and persists throughout every point of the sales call. A probe can be a basic question:

> "What treatment options do you generally consider?"

or based on past experience:

> "In the past you indicated that you tend to refer these patients out to physical therapy."

or presumptive:

> "It must be getting more difficult to choose a treatment option in light of the recent warnings on the use of NSAIDs for patients who have had or are at risk of heart disease or stroke. What are your other options?"

The presumptive statement allows you to control the conversation. For instance, consider a doctor who utilizes physical therapy as a first choice. This doctor will reasonably assume that you are there to substitute your services for physical therapy. The doctor may choose to not mention physical therapy as his first choice, and then may protect his choice by deflecting the conversation to medication. Assuming that you have sold persuasively against medication and the doctor gives every indication that he buys into what you are saying, you should see patients in a relatively short period of time. If it has been 3 months and you have yet to see a patient, either this doctor didn't buy in to your presentation but said he did (see the section titled "The 'Yes' Doctor" in Chapter 4) or the doctor is not being straightforward. You need to move the selling process forward, especially when you know there are patients who could benefit from your care. A presumptive statement in this situation might sound like this:

> "Doctor, it seems we have been focusing on NSAIDs, yet they aren't the only criterion. I am sure you have patients you have referred for physical therapy. How do you discriminate between medication and physical therapy for your patients?"

Probing questions are fun. It is a rewarding situation to break through barriers that then allow a doctor to open up and really tell you about what he or she likes about a first choice and areas that he or she doesn't like or wishes could be improved. You can investigate as deep as you want; just make sure the doctor isn't becoming protective or offended by your line of questioning. There are proper ways of wording questions and improper ways that can be a source of aggravation to the doctor. Do ask the doctor:

> "How do you decide between medication and physical therapy for a patient with lower back pain?"

Don't follow a doctor's reply with, "Why?" The word *why* alone is adversarial. Do ask the doctor:

> "What problems do you encounter when referring patients to physical therapy?" or "What side effects does the patient complain about when taking medications?"

Ask probes and direct the attention if possible to the area that you think will help you illustrate why manipulation and chiropractic care might be a better choice for this doctor's patients.

Seeds of Doubt

These are planted by the opening statement, but they can also be utilized as a probe. If you know the doctor uses NSAIDs, you could create a seed of doubt in your opening statement:

> "Doctor, for patients who have a tendency for GI issues, prescribing NSAIDs for their back pain must by tricky."

In this case you are identifying a specific patient who won't be a candidate for the doctor's first choice and you are instead paving the path to insert chiropractic services as an alternate. It is the first step toward changing the physician's treatment habits.

Features and Benefits

When discussing the features and benefits of chiropractic care, you are not only explaining what the results are for manipulation but also why they are important. For instance:

> "Patients with recurrent lower back pain in this 2-week to 48-month follow-up study with almost 3,000 patients enjoyed the same rapid decline in pain as the medical patients who were mostly treated with medication. Chiropractic care is less invasive than medication, so if a patient has a risk for or sensitivity to medications, chiropractic care could provide the same results while avoiding medication." (Show Figure 5 of the study titled "A Practice-Based Study of Patients with Acute and Chronic Low Back Pain Attending Primary Care and Chiropractic Physicians: Two-Week to 48-Month Follow-Up" by Mitchell Haas et al.)[1]

Features and benefits can also consist of a "meet and beat." When promoting a study, you will utilize research to prove that chiropractic care is at least as effective if not more effective than the competition, and then you beat the competition by stating the advantages chiropractic has over the doctor's first-line treatment option and your competition. When you "meet" the competition, you are illustrating that your services can meet the efficacy or safety level that the doctor likes about his current therapeutic choice. When you "beat" the competition, you are indicating that you can solve or improve upon what the doctor dislikes about his current therapeutic choice.

It is more than likely that doctors will try to punch a few holes in your information by throwing up a few more objections. That is a normal part of the sales process; don't freeze up, just keep clarifying and referring to the literature. Use your probes to uncover why the question is being asked. If the doctor states that he or she feels exercise is better than manipulation, you need to clarify that statement to uncover his or her position and an angle on how you can meet and beat. For example, does the doctor prefer exercise because it is active care? Is exercise preferred because it is strengthening in nature and therefore likely to prevent more recurrences? Once you get past the objections and gain commitment that he or she likes the treatment response illustrated in the clinical study, you can then move into the "beat" section of the call.

> "Doctor, you indicated that it often takes 5 or 6 days for your patients to secure a first physical therapy treatment appointment. This means that not only are patients not resuming activities of daily living, but they also become more and more difficult to treat. For patients who might be on disability, the sooner they can receive care, the sooner they will be back at work and not on disability. I recognize this need and I take patients on a walk-in basis or by appointment within 24 hours of their first call. This means less disability paperwork for you, and your patients will be happier with your ability to send them somewhere they don't have to wait for insurance preauthorizations and clearance. Would that be beneficial?"

This is a great example of why you gather information with probes prior to the presentation of data. If you encounter a doctor who really wants to stick with the primary treatment of physical therapy, and you already showed a very valid proof source that manipulation is more efficacious than physical therapy, this doctor is more than likely going to start throwing up some walls to protect his or her first-line therapy. If you had not already uncovered the fact that the doctor is dissatisfied with the wait time and you asked that same question, the doctor would probably tell you he or she didn't experience any delays with appointments as a means of protecting this first choice of therapy.

Trial Closing

Checking in with the doctor on what he or she thinks about the information you are presenting is considered a trial closing. In the previous example, you would trial close by asking the following:

> "Would it be a valuable service for your patients to be able to leave your practice and walk into my clinic to immediately begin treatment for their back pain?"

You should check in with the doctor after every important point to determine what the buy-in is, and if he or she isn't buying it, ask for clarification. In the preceding example, a doctor could say no, which has several different meanings:

- No, that is not what I expect—these numbers are much better!
- No, I think physical therapy has better rates. [Two things are possibly going on here: (1) The doctor is providing a false objection either because he or she hasn't yet bought in to the mechanism of action for manipulation or still has an unvoiced barrier present in accepting chiropractic. (2) It could be your approach. It is possible that the doctor felt you bashed his or her primary therapeutic choice. This second objection is one of the most difficult to battle and you must tread lightly. Remember Sales Rule 5? When in trouble, ask a clarifying question. "Doctor, could you clarify for me what you would expect to see in the outcome assessment?" Perhaps the doctor misunderstood the rates, perhaps it is the study design that he or she disagrees with; you won't know unless you ask the clarifying questions.]

If you have a home run clinical and you know it is solid, something else is brewing. You have to start taking some backward steps. Once you get the doctor to clarify the objection, you may be able to back up and cover it using the same study or you may need to pull out another study to overcome the objection. As you can see, the conversational approach allows you to step back and forth in the process and back and forth in the material. If you know your research, you can do this with ease.

Closing the Doctor

In this portion of the sales call, you summarize the pertinent points of the call, reminding the doctor that he or she agreed to efficacy/safety/and or cost as well as why chiropractic might be a better choice as a result of some advantage over the competition, so that you can then ask for referrals. We touched briefly on this in the main steps of the sales process model. Let's develop the point a little further. I am not a huge fan of an action close and really utilized it only once or twice in my career. An action close can be very cheesy:

Bad Action Close:

"Doctor, do I have your commitment that you will refer your next 20 back pain patients to me?"

Yuck! The doctor will not like it either. You just went from professional doctor having a professional dialogue to cheap car salesperson.

Presumptive Close:

If you just spent 20 minutes going over material and tying it in with a patient type, covered managed care, overcame the objections, and have the doctor's buy-in, I think it is okay to presume you have the doctor's business, in which case I recommend the following type of close:

"Doctor, I look forward to working with you and helping your patients with chronic lower back pain."

or

"Doctor, based on this information, would you have any hesitation in referring a recurrent lower back pain patient to my office for chiropractic services?"

If you feel that you hit a home run in your conversation with the doctor and then you fail to see any patients, your follow-up calls will have to be more pointed and direct in your promotional efforts.

"Doctor, in our last meeting you seemed very interested in the data illustrating the success of manipulation in treating recurrent lower back pain; however, I have not had the opportunity to see your patients. Do you have any further questions that I can help answer or that are preventing you from referring patients over to my office?"

Some personality types, which I will discuss later, need a friendly nudge. In the preceding example, perhaps the doctor responds that he or she hasn't referred any patients because of insurance. Perhaps in your enthusiasm you forgot to cover this point, or perhaps it was bad luck that the first patient the doctor referred had an insurance plan you aren't on. In this case, you might respond:

"Doctor, you indicated that Lifeguard is a very small portion of your managed care profile. I don't take Lifeguard, but I would be more than happy to refer you to a colleague who does. Just as a reminder, I do take Blue Cross/Blue Shield, and if I am correct that constitutes almost half of your patient base. Is that correct? Great, when you look at the out-of-pocket expenses for Blue Cross/Blue Shield, you will see that for chiropractic services the patient can expect a $10 copay after meeting the medical deductible of $100."

After clarifying the reason for nonreferrals and perhaps reminding the doctor of the findings from the previous presentation, you will have to again await any referrals. If they still don't come, it is time to take a direct and friendly approach and decide if this doctor is worth your time:

"Doctor, I have presented data relevant to chronic recurrent lower back pain patients to you twice and both times you received the information well, but you have yet to refer any patients. What treatments have you utilized instead of chiropractic care for your more recent back pain patients that you felt were not compatible for chiropractic care?"

Perhaps you haven't demonstrated the right competitor. Probing questions and clarifying questions will eventually provide an answer or a gut instinct that this particular doctor just isn't going to refer to you and is uncomfortable telling you why. If this happens, move on and perhaps just stay in contact by letter when more recent research comes out. Over time the physician's feelings may change.

Remember to carry the patient picture throughout your sales call. It is much more memorable to the doctor to think of a specific patient type in his or her practice and apply your solution to it.

The "I Don't Like Chiropractic" Response

It might happen that you introduce yourself and the doctor says, "I don't like chiropractors." From a dignity standpoint alone, how do you respond? Try the following response and keep in mind the fact that you have won over many patients who didn't think you were going to help them either.

"I am sorry to hear that you feel that way, and I understand that in the past my profession has made some claims that might make you leery. However, the chiropractic profession has made great strides in scientific research and has shown itself to be effective in the eyes of managed care, the military, and most important much of the community we live and practice in. Perhaps you might be interested in knowing how I treat patients as a chiropractor and my educational background so that if you have a patient that comes in and tells you he or she is seeing a chiropractor for lower back pain you can understand from where some of the benefits might arise."

At this point, you either have the doctor or you don't. You either will get a begrudging sigh of "go ahead and tell me," or you will still have the door slammed on you. If the door is slammed, you need to put on your emotional rubber suit and let it bounce off of you. It is very likely it isn't you but rather a doctor who has no bedside manner or desire to change habits. Why would you want to develop professional rapport with this type of physician? If your pride and dignity can't get over it, leave information with the front desk, and if you want to try to win over the doctor with kindness, leave information with a snack or drink that the staff knows he or she might like. At least you got your message through somehow.

Selling to a physician should take you out of your comfort level . . . at first. This isn't a one-time sell. It is one that should continue to form a growing professional relationship—one that will allow you to constantly expand what type of referrals you might expect by always presenting new and pertinent information. With the amount of research currently available and more on its way, you won't run out of material.

Postcall Notes

When you leave the physician's office, you should create some sort of file, paper or electronic, that reflects your call. You should indicate which study you discussed, what the doctor's reaction was, any office stats or competitive information you received, and clinical rationale. *Most important, you should note what your immediate gut instinct is for the next call objective and what information you should present at that time.* You may think that you will remember the call verbatim; however, that is your adrenaline talking. I constantly referred to my postcall notes to follow up with the doctor, which reminded me of what information I had already supplied and allowed me to remember what worked and what didn't work with that personality. Please take 5 minutes to write your notes immediately after your meeting. The longer you wait, the more of the little details you will forget.

Marketing Ethics

It seems that every aspect of health care has rules and regulations. Marketing is no different, and marketing specifically to physicians comes with its own special set of laws. The two laws to be concerned with are Stark law and the Federal Anti-kickback law. What I have listed here are the highlights and my own interpretation drawn from my experience and knowledge from pharmaceutical sales as well as common sense. If there is any gray area that you experience, you should consult an attorney. I am not an attorney and neither is this text intended as a substitute for legal advice; it is just a guideline.

Stark Law

Stark law is also known as the Physician Self-Referral Statute. Although there are many components to it, I cover only the portion related to marketing. In essence, Stark law comes into play when you promote to a physician. Anything of value, "food, paying for dinner and gifts," falls under the category of "monetary value." Stark law was created to prevent medical doctors from referring patients for any service (medical or diagnostic) or prescribing medication in exchange for something of monetary value if the doctor or any immediate relative has an interest in the place or physician he or she is referring patients to. The concept here is pretty obvious, and it is designed to protect consumers and avoid insurance fraud. A referral in its entirety should purely be for the benefit of the patient. A few years ago, many of our prime-time networks produced stories, most of which were centered around the pharmaceutical industry, that showed medical physicians being wined and dined at five-star restaurants, enjoying spa treatments, playing golf, and staying at resorts to elicit prescriptions for their product. This is now taboo. In fact, anything that even remotely "resembles or appears" to be extravagant is a no-no.

As a profession, chiropractors have endured enough bad press, most of it unwarranted. We all know that the media can take one or two cases as an example and sensationalize them so that they negatively affect the entire profession. Keep this in mind as you entertain your physicians. Money does not have to be exchanged for something to be considered of monetary value; gifts and excessive entertaining are also considered monetary. The total amount of food and gifts should not exceed more than approximately $300 annually per doctor.

The second example of monetary gifts are ones of substance. Some gifts pharmaceutical reps used to give out were textbooks, ICD-9 books, and subscriptions to journals. The new rule that I worked under limited gifts to a $100 cap per physician per year. This meant that if I gave a doctor a book valued at $99, that doctor was off limits to any other representative in my company to receive further gifts, and these data were tracked. When I submitted the expense form, I had to allocate my company's identification number for the doctor and the doctor's address. Once this hit the databases, no other gifts could be applied for this doctor. This prevented two reps from the same company purchasing a $200 book and splitting the cost between each other's budget. As you probably know, it is very difficult to purchase most medical textbooks for under $100. In addition, all gifts must be educational in nature and related to the class of drugs being represented. For instance, sending flowers was not educational and was not appropriate; in fact doing so would more than likely result in termination. Selling an antidepressant and purchasing the doctor an automatic blood pressure cuff was also not allowed.

What can you do to entertain doctors and help them understand your area of expertise? There are several available options. The first is lunch. Bring them a modest lunch, spending no more than $10 to $12 per person including meal, drink, and dessert. If you are going out to dinner, keep your cost to no more than $100 per person, and this includes appetizers, salad, entrée, dinner, dessert, and drinks. Not only does this maintain compliance, but it also keeps your costs from skyrocketing. Most doctors are aware of these guidelines, but because you are a doctor they may not realize it applies in the same manner. You can simply tell the doctor this a promotional dinner and the Stark law applies. If that is not enough explanation, you might want to reconsider forging a professional relationship. I can already hear, "Yes, but what if we are good friends already?" or "Who is going to catch us?" I can't answer that for you because it is a legal question, but I can advise you that it is the "appearance" that matters, and the stakes are too high for the entire profession to even consider deviating from such a strict line of professional conduct.

For more information on the Stark law, please contact your local state chiropractic association prior to purchasing any promotional items or entertaining.

Federal Anti-Kickback Law

The law known as the anti-kickback law centers around federally funded programs such as Medicare and Medicaid. The anti-kickback law provides both criminal and civil penalties for individuals and entities that knowingly offer, pay, solicit, or receive bribes or kickbacks or other remuneration to induce business reimbursable by Medicare, Medicaid, or other governmental programs.

The anti-kickback law is very similar to the Stark law but focuses on Medicare and Medicaid. Any violation by any involved party can be cause for civil and criminal legal recourse. Stark law only allows for a civil legal recourse.

There are many important factors associated with promoting to physicians, and it is important to be aware of them. Ignorance is not an excuse!

REFERENCE

1. Haas M, Goldberg B, Aickin M, Ganger B, Attwood M. A practice-based study of patients with acute and chronic low back pain attending primary care and chiropractic physicians: Two-week to 48-month follow-up. *J Manipulative Physiol Ther.* 2004; 27:160–169.

Chapter 4

Selling to Different Personalities

I n sales training, a fair amount of focus is placed on presenting material to different personality types. Modifying your approach based on personalities will affect your presentation for two primary reasons:

1. Personalities respond to different sales aids. Some personalities respond to the glossy, colorful charts that make up the master visual aid (MVA). Some prefer clinical studies. Others don't necessarily have a preference as long as the information is reputable.

2. Personalities have different motives for changing referral habits. Doctors are motivated to change their referral habits for various reasons. Some refer based on the literature, whereas others refer based on what will make their patients happy.

In our everyday life as chiropractors, we deal with an astounding number of personalities exhibited by our patients. As you go through your day treating patients, you exhibit several different approaches to these patients with the primary goal of helping them with their condition and winning them over as consumers. All chiropractors have had a patient snap at the front desk because they had to fill out paperwork. The majority of these patients were in pain. Chiropractors excel at turning these patients around by observing the patient and adapting their approach to the patient's needs. In that way, adapting your approach and presentation to the medical community will be quite similar.

When it comes to patients, we all have those who we enjoy seeing and those who we don't. In such situations, most patients move on to find a doctor more suited to their personality; unfortunately others don't! It can be the same in sales. Identify several doctors with whom you can develop professional rapport and work with them.

WIFM (pronounced "wif-em") stands for What's in It for Me? When you sell, you want to think about how WIFM applies to the doctor's practice, patients, and personality. In other words, what is the physician's need that you can solve with chiropractic?

Personality Categories

People respond to different styles of speaking, so much so that many books have been written on the matter. If you speak fast, you will tend to tune out people who speak slowly or in a monotone. In fact, if you speak and think quickly, you probably notice that when you take a patient's history who speaks slowly and monotonously that you have to utilize more patience and more focus. Likewise, a doctor who is clinically minded and speaks slowly and deliberately can be overwhelmed by a fast-paced loud patient or sales approach.

The main personality categories are meant to be a general guide. Certainly, every doctor is capable of having a mixture or a combination of different personalities, but there will be one that dominates.

1. The Authoritative Doctor
2. The Pleaser Doctor
3. The Introverted Doctor
4. The Fun Doctor
5. The Needy Doctor
6. The "Yes" Doctor

If you are outgoing and you sell to an outgoing doctor, make sure you remember to sell and not just make a great friend. A great friend and colleague does not guarantee referrals. Take the following example into consideration. When I was in sales training, one of my instructors indicated that he had a friend who was a "fun" doctor and who was also on his call panel when he was a sales rep. He presumed that because they were friends that the doctor would automatically write his product. This was back in the day when you could really wine and dine a doctor. Eventually, the sales rep's manager asked him to explain why he was spending so much of the budget on a doctor who was proving to be a poor return on investment (which is manager code for "what are you doing wrong in your sales approach?"). So, the instructor asked his doctor friend why he wasn't prescribing his product. His doctor friend responded that he knew nothing about the drug. He didn't know the dosage, the formulary (insurance benefit for pharmaceuticals have different priorities on different insurance formularies; as such one drug may enjoy open access on one insurance plan and require extra approval processes on another insurance formulary), the indication, so he just didn't bother to prescribe it. The lesson here is to make sure that you are always educating your physicians on the importance of chiropractic manipulation whether or not you develop a social relationship with them, too.

When you evaluate a physician you may call on, the front desk is a great source of information. Ask pointed questions that may reveal the doctor's personality so that you have some information on what you can present. Possible questions include these:

Does the doctor subscribe to many journals? Which ones?

Does the doctor attend seminars? More than the average doctor?

Does the doctor spend a lot of time out of the office playing sports, going to concerts, going to the symphony, eating out?

Does the doctor do a lot of speaking engagements?

Does the doctor stay late at night making phone calls, or does the doctor tend to run late with appointments?

These questions can yield insight into their personalities, For instance a doctor who subscribes to multiple journals is obviously intently interested in research.

A doctor doesn't necessarily have to fall into one personality category and may in fact have traits of one or more personality types. The question is, which one is the strongest component? For instance, a doctor may exhibit a trait of an egomaniac doctor but also show signs of being introverted. Which type seems dominant? Your gut instinct will be the best judge. Being well prepared and having the ability to mirror voice inflections and manners will allow you to be successful with all personality types.

The Authoritative Doctor

The doctors who most frequently exhibit this personality trait tend to be

Heads of clinics

Specialists including neurologists, orthopedic surgeons, cardiologists, and oncologists

These doctors tend to have a large ego. The ego may not always be bad, but it does mean they have a tremendous amount of confidence, so the material you present should be compelling. These doctors tend to be brief, direct, and to the point. They can be charming or they can be abrasive. They don't always let you know you "sold" them, but they won't hesitate to tell you why you are wrong. Authoritative doctors are great for the selling process in that they have no problem offering an objection and they are quick decision makers. It can be difficult to be brief with a study that has a lot of pertinent information, but you should pick the main benefits of the study and leave the little things out for this personality type.

Sales Aids

The MVA is the best aid to start with because you need to be quick. However, these doctors are equally capable of getting into a clinical if they have the time and the interest in what you are presenting. Some like to "tell you" and "teach" you what they will do, so taking a sales approach that is "curious" about their thoughts on back pain and the associated treatments allows them to educate you while you gather information. Don't mistake *curious* for the need to present in a timid voice. Although you need to ask questions that allow the doctor to educate you, it is still desirable for you to use voice inflection that implies confidence. When it comes to your turn to educate on chiropractic manipulation, this is especially true. In addition, if you disagree with this doctor because you know without a doubt that you have the supporting material to prove your point, you should "politely" disagree. This doctor will respect your viewpoint if you can confidently, properly, and concisely illustrate your point through credible research.

Selling Style

These are "bottom line" doctors. *Bottom line* means that you need to have a clear, concise message with no filler. These doctors will be direct, they tend to presume that you have a sales point in mind, and they usually accurately guess what it is. As such, they tend to skip right to the point and offer what it is they like or don't like. They tend not to lie just to get you out of their office, and they appreciate a direct and honest response. You will not cover an entire research article unless they guide you through it. You may walk in and think you are presenting lower back and find out on the spot that you will be presenting the neck because that is the information they want to see.

The key with these doctors is organization as well as using a direct and self-assured manner. You should have the information readily available for almost any of the key topics and maintain a sense of calmness without being a pushover. Confidence in your data is a key issue. This will not likely be a long presentation, and doctors may request information and ask that you leave it. They will probably read it, and this is a good reason to schedule a follow-up lunch or meeting to see what they thought of it. If they didn't read it, when you return on a future date you can probably detail the study to them and they will be more open to it because they know they requested it, and they requested it because they were truly interested in the topic.

The doctor will either say it looks good, ask more questions, or offer an objection. He or she may also not have time at that moment to comment, so ask her for a time to come back and ask what material he or she would like to hear about (neck, lower back, headaches). Ask whether there is any particular head-to-head study he or she might find interesting when you return.

Whereas you always want to be concise with this personality type, don't be so brief that you don't relay the information. Remember, this doctor requires you to use a confident, authoritative tone as you present the information. Weakness or timidness on your part implies weakness of your material. At the same time, you need to balance the sell by allowing the doctor to make the decisions and "educate" you. The WIFM for this doctor is to provide the most up-to-date therapeutic treatment choices and the scientific treatment rationale to support the choice.

The Pleaser Doctor

These doctors go out of their way to help their patients. The selling features to them relate 100% to the effect the treatment will have on the patients. This type of doctor most closely resembles many chiropractors, family practitioners, and doctors of osteopathy. These doctors take a lot of time with patients, and they feel bad if they leave the office without returning all the calls themselves the same day they received their messages. They wage the fight for insurance and preauthorizations; and they follow a patient's care even when they refer them out. They spend a lot of time with patient families when a situation warrants it. They research alternative means of treatments when the ordinary doesn't work. They tend to enjoy high patient satisfaction and loyalty. Working as a team with this physician is key. It shouldn't take too much of your time to maintain the team by providing a quick telephone update or brief written report—all they want to know is that you have seen the patient and are taking the lead to provide care. They will respond to the patient satisfaction data that chiropractors have; they will appreciate the hands-on approach, the ability to get patients into care immediately, the length of time that you take with each patient, and the personal service you are willing to provide to their patients. These points are the WIFM for these doctors.

> *Sales aids:* Either the MVA or clinical will do based on time. As with any sales encounter, you should have both and watch for the doctor's reaction to the material.
>
> *Selling style:* Use a warm, direct, compassionate approach. Do not mistake these doctors as pushovers, though.

The Introverted Doctor

The introverted doctor is typically a very quiet person who finds most forms of sales obnoxious. Therefore, for this personality type a truly educational approach that dives deep into the research is best. Introverted doctors may take longer to answer your probing questions because they carefully consider the question and their answer. They tend to avoid eye contact, and they can be friendly, but they tend not to discuss personal aspects of their life with you when asked. Therefore, spend only a fraction of your time socializing with this doctor. If you see his or her office or observe the clinical surroundings, you will notice many journals; introverted doctors tend to have a "professor's" desk, meaning they have piles of paperwork and they may even seem disorganized. This type of doctor responds well to clinical reprints and does not like a glossy MVA simply because of its "glitz." This doctor can get into the nuts and bolts of the clinical or may offer you very little feedback and just take it all in. He may or may not refute the information even if he doesn't like it to avoid any type of "selling" by you. He may give you an indication of his buy-in without meaning to, such as a crinkled eyebrow that suggests disagreement, or a very subtle nod of the head. I once announced to this type of doctor with a smile on my face that I noticed he was wrinkling his eyebrows. It was enough to get him to admit that he disagreed with my data, and we were able to have a quick laugh and conversation about it.

The introverted doctor is heavily into research and clinical information. Typically, when you sell to these doctors you can use a quieter voice, socialize less, and can constantly gauge their buy-in on the information that you are presenting either through observation or by asking. The WIFM for these doctors is a solid and reputable evidence-based option for treatment for their patients. Because they are very familiar with clinicals, you can probably go into detail on the study design and setup. Using research terms is effective, and this doctor type will easily understand the methods as well as the reasons why studies that examine physical treatments are difficult to blind. These doctors will be interested in the mechanism of manipulation. They readily absorb data, so once they get it, they retain it. Being forceful and aggressive with this type of doctor is ineffective as is being overly social. This is a great doctor to take out to dinner with a thought leader in your community, such as a chiropractic professor or another clinically minded doctor, and ask questions that create communication with the two doctors on the research surrounding manipulation.

> *Sales aids:* Prefers clinical papers. Of any group, this type is more likely to accept a broader range of studies, provided the methodology holds up.

Selling style: Use a more scientifically oriented, more in-depth style focused on the mechanism of action for manipulation.

The Fun Doctor

This is a doctor who, although fun, can be very exasperating to sell to, especially if you are an introverted authoritative doctor type. The key here is to be brief, fun, engaging, and patient. This doctor will be fun but all over the place. He or she would rather talk to you more about current events than about your information. These types respond better to glossy graphs rather than clinical studies. They are difficult to sell to because it is hard to keep their attention. For these doctors, the WIFM is in explaining how excited their patients will be about less-invasive techniques that can help them with their back pain. These doctors tend to be easy to get out for dinner; just make sure you are selling while you develop this professional relationship.

The key is to express the appreciation their patients will feel for the referral while emphasizing the fact that you will also be making the doctor's job easier and without complications.

Sales aids: MVA

Selling style: The patient type should be brief: "Chronic lower back pain patients."

The Needy Doctor

This is a doctor who will require the most time and will always be testing you to see how far you are willing to extend yourself. Realize that there is a difference between providing a service that is appreciated by the doctor and being made to jump through unnecessary hoops to earn appreciation. If the doctor has a big practice, you might think it is worth it. Most of us don't have much patience for this type of personality in general. The loyalties from this doctor are completely related to how far and how high you are willing to jump, and that isn't conducive to developing professional rapport. Making matters worse is that their requests tend to be redundant and needless. They aren't clingy; they just enjoy the show of watching everyone around them cater to their needs. My advice is to move on unless the results are well worth it and the requests are reasonable. It is better to develop a relationship with two or three smaller practices and cut a needy big fish loose. For chiropractors who are mostly the pleaser personality, be cautious of a needy doctor.

The Yes Doctor

Many times doctors will respond positively to your sales approach and say they "love" your product, that the information is strong, and then they do nothing with it. This is a promotional nightmare. You aren't creating a relationship with these doctors: These doctors are either too nice to tell you why they don't like chiropractic care, or they don't like to be sold to, so they say they love your product in an effort to stop the sales process. A proper way to approach this problem is to ask the doctors where they think manipulation might be successful in comparison to where they find your competitors to be successful. These doctors may also be what can be referred to as "spreaders," meaning they will send two or three patients your way, and then send two or three patients to physical therapy, and so on.

Fast and Slow Adopters

People in general have a tendency to either hear about something and immediately decide whether they like it or not, while others can take months to cautiously make their decisions. They are frequently referred to as fast adopters and slow adopters. Doctors who are buying your information may need time and multiple conversations to decide if chiropractic services are truly an option for their patients, and even then begin slowly with their referrals. Slow adopters may be confused with a "yes" doctor, and your instinct will be the best guide to determining the reason you may not be seeing immediate referrals.

There are pros and cons to both types of adopters. For slow adopters the benefit is that once you have them it is difficult for any competitor to sway them away form their decision; the con is that it takes a while to earn their referrals. Fast adopters are great for earning immediate business if you hit on the information that means something to them; at the same time their con is that a persuasive competitor can easily switch them over to their service or product.

Fun and authoritative doctors tend to be fast adopters (or decide quickly not to be adopters at all). While introverted and pleaser doctors may be slow adopters, pushing a slow adopter to make a decision is not a good idea; rather take the time to foster the relationship and trust.

Examples of Dialogue for Different Personalities

The following provides a general idea on how you might phrase similar questions to different types of personalities. It also provides different sales angles that you can utilize to grab their attention based on their personalities. This is not meant to be a strict dialogue but rather to illustrate the difference in approach that you should consider using for different personalities.

In each of these examples I have used a patient with chronic lower back pain who is no longer suitable for nonsteroidal anti-inflammatory drug (NSAID) therapy due to the new American Heart Association's (AHA) warning.[1] In addition, I have created a doctor who prescribes medications first and physical therapy second. When referring to physical therapists, this doctor likes active exercises. Your objective is to take the place of the physical therapy referral for these patients no longer suitable for NSAIDs by offering exercises and manipulation. First you want to establish that the doctor is aware of the new warnings; then you want to find out the clinical rationale for how he or she recommends treatments.

There are many studies that could be utilized to demonstrate the efficacy of manipulation for lower back pain; the one you choose will either be to prove efficacy compared to NSAIDs or to compare how manipulation compares to physical therapy. How you choose which one to present will be the doctor's response or simply by instinct. The study is not discussed here, but for demonstration purposes in the closing section, I utilize numbers and comments that reference the UK BEAM study, which we will go over later. Each study that is discussed in this book will point out pertinent features and graphs as well as provide you with "bottom line" statements. For now let's focus on verbiage as it relates to personalities.

Opening Statements with a Seed of Doubt

Authoritative Doctor: Patients with lower back pain that is not resolving on its own must be difficult to treat if they have or are at risk of heart disease in light of the AHA's new warnings on NSAID use. (Direct, presumptive, to the point)

Pleaser Doctor: The new AHA warnings on the use of NSAIDs must make treating lower back pain patients at risk of heart disease or stroke very difficult, especially if their back pain prevents them from their activities of daily living. (Sympathetic)

Introverted Doctor: The AHA has posted new recommendations for patients at risk or who have heart disease and the use of NSAIDs; for your back pain patients this means finding a new therapy that has been established in research to be effective. (Science based)

Fun Doctor: Patients who have chronic lower back pain can be difficult to treat, especially with the new warnings on NSAIDs by the AHA for those at risk or who have heart disease. (Problem oriented from the doctor's perspective)

Probes

Authoritative Doctor: What other options do you consider for managing their back pain?

Pleaser Doctor: What other treatment options do you consider in lieu of medication to help decrease their pain and improve their quality of life?

Introverted Doctor: How do you decide new treatment options for these patients?

Fun Doctor: What are your other options that you choose from?

Follow-up Probes (note the sympathetic statement at the beginning of each sentence)

Authoritative Doctor: That makes perfect sense. When you refer to physical therapy, are you looking for active care or therapeutic modalities? Do you find that patients must wait a long time for their first appointment? Are you familiar with the evidence-based research for chiropractic manipulation compared to exercises?

Pleaser Doctor: I understand and am sure your patients have enjoyed some great results. Do you feel they get the most out of active exercises or therapeutic modalities? Do you find that patients must wait a long time for their first appointment? What amount of time are you spending on preauthorizations? (Note: A pleaser doctor might not feel that this is a problem, but given a choice any doctor and their staff would be thrilled to limit the need for preauthorizations. If the doctor says it is not a problem, you can relate it back to the delay in treatment while waiting for the insurance company to grant the authorization.) Evidence-based research for chiropractic manipulation has resulted in very positive findings and high rates of patient satisfaction. Have you had the opportunity to review some of the research especially comparing manipulation and exercises?

Introverted Doctor: That is a great clinical rationale. When you refer to physical therapy for a chronic patient, do you feel that exercises or therapeutic modalities should be the primary focus? There is a lot of evidence-based research on lower back pain. Are you familiar with the research focused on chiropractic manipulation and the positive findings on lower back pain compared to back pain treated with exercise?

Fun Doctor: I understand. Are you finding that you are now faced with higher numbers of preauthorizations for physical therapy? It must be frustrating for you and your patients to wait a couple of weeks for treatment to commence. Do you feel that physical therapy for chronic back pain should consist of therapeutic modalities or active exercises? Have you seen the current research validating the efficacy of manipulation for lower back pain compared to exercises?

Now is when you would refer to a study and educate the physician on the study design, set up, and conclusions. If time does not allow, at least provide them with a bottom line statement of the study.

Close

Authoritative Doctor: Doctor, do you feel that these results in favor of manipulation over exercises or at least in combination with exercise make manipulation a viable and noninvasive option for patients with lower back pain who can no longer take NSAIDs? (Assumes that at some point you mentioned that chiropractors are specialists in manipulation and that you illustrated that manipulation provided the most efficacy.)

Pleaser Doctor: Doctor, the 1,334 patients in this study had a more robust response to care and were out of pain faster, allowing them to resume their daily activities. We also discussed that chiropractors offer safe and competent chiropractic manipulation in addition to standard physical therapy care. For patients who have a contraindication to NSAID use, do you feel that manipulation offers a safe alternative to medication and would help resolve their pain faster? (Assumes that you illustrated the safety of chiropractic manipulation and that you can still offer the other physical therapy options this doctor prefers. Also, it assumes that you are willing to take walk-in referrals.)

Introverted Doctor: Doctor, this is compelling research with statistically significant findings in favor of manipulation over exercise. Do you feel chiropractic manipulation might also benefit your patients? (Assumes that you illustrated the net benefit of manipulation to be more statistically significant in the UK BEAM trial.)[2]

Fun Doctor: Doctor, do you feel that the outcomes from this large population study are reflective of how chiropractic manipulation would help solve your problem with these at-risk patients and at the same time make your patients appreciative of your fast resolution for their condition? (Assumes that you took the burden of performing any preauthorizations and provide immediate access to care.)

Conclusion

As you form more relationships in the medical community, make sure you keep personalities in mind as you invite doctors to dinner. Inviting a social doctor out with a research doctor will be irritating for both as will inviting the director type out with the relating type. They are all motivated by different approaches and have different bedside manners and styles of communication and interaction.

Selling to doctors involves adjusting to their needs and presenting data such that the information fits their needs and expectations. If you think that you have no experience in sales, think again; you do it every day with your patients. This sales model is just that: A model to work with as you get started. Ultimately, you will find the doctors with whom you want to forge relationships, and you will develop an educational sales approach that works for that purpose. You can never go wrong in making an earnest effort to bring doctors a treatment option that can benefit their patients, especially if you promote with integrity and respect.

References

1. Antman EM, Bennett JS, Daugherty A, Furberg C, Roberts H, Taubert KA. Use of non-steroidal anti-inflammatory drugs. An update for clinicians. A scientific statement from the American Heart Association. *Circulation*. 2007:115(12):1634–1642.
2. UK Back Pain Exercise and Manipulation (UK BEAM) Trial Team. UK Back pain Exercise and Manipulation (UK BEAM) trial—national randomized trial of physical treatments for back pain in primary care: objectives, design and interventions. *BMC Health Serv Res*. 2003;3:13. Available at http://www.biomedcentral.com/1472-6963/3/16. Accessed January 8, 2008.

Chapter 5

Knowing Your Target Audience

When placing your product in the marketplace, you have to know where your product or service falls compared to your competitors'. (We examine competitors later in the book.) It is also critical to know who you are selling to and their desire to know about your service. In the case of chiropractic and the treatment of lower back, neck, and headaches, what are the current treatment guidelines for medical doctors? What do medical doctors think about chiropractors, and what objections can we expect?

Do Doctors Want to Know About Chiropractic Services?

Yes! Doctors are responding to consumer demand for alternative health care that replaces medication and in some cases the need for surgery. Certainly, they must feel the overwhelming obligation to treat a patient with back pain with something other than nonsteroidal anti-inflammatory drugs (NSAIDs). Not only are consumers demanding alternatives, but warnings and side effects plague what was once touted as a benign class of drugs such as NSAIDs.[1] There are some interesting data on what doctors think of chiropractic.

"Referral Patterns and Attitudes of Primary Care Physicians Towards Chiropractors." Barry R. Greene, Monica Smith, Veerasathpurush Allareddy, and Mitchell Haas. *BMC Complementary and Alternative Medicine.* 2006;6:5.

Abstract

Background: Despite the increasing usage and popularity of chiropractic care, there has been limited research conducted to examine the professional relationships between conventionally trained primary care physicians (PCPs) and chiropractors (DCs). The objectives of our study were to contrast the intra-professional referral patterns among PCPs with referral patterns to DCs, and to identify predictors of PCP referral to DCs.

Methods: We mailed a survey instrument to all practicing PCPs in the state of Iowa. Descriptive statistics were used to summarize their responses. Multivariable logistic regression analyses were conducted to identify demographic factors associated with inter-professional referral behaviors.

Results: A total of 517 PCPs (33%) participated in the study. PCPs enjoyed strong intraprofessional referral relationships with other PCPs. Although patients exhibited a great deal of interest in chiropractic care, PCPs were unlikely themselves to make formal referral relationships with DCs. PCPs in a private practice arrangement were more likely to exhibit positive referral attitudes towards DCs ($p = 0.01$).

Conclusion: PCPs enjoy very good professional relationships with other PCPs. However, the lack of direct formalized referral relationships between PCPs and chiropractors has implications for efficiency, continuity, quality, and patient safety in the health care delivery system. Future research must focus on identifying facilitators and barriers for developing positive relationships between PCPs and chiropractors.

This study, published in 2006, is a look at 517 Iowa-based physicians, specifically 404 medical doctors and 109 doctors of osteopathy.[2] Together they represent 33% of the entire medical professionals in this statewide survey. Doctors were asked questions relating to several topics, some of which are specifically outlined below. Not only does this study illustrate where chiropractors stand in the medical community, but it also provides a baseline to measure future studies against. It also tells us who might be the most appropriate providers to start promoting to.

Referral Patterns

According to this study, when an allopathic doctor refers to another allopathic provider, the doctors initiated the referral approximately 99% of the time.[2] However when they referred the patient to a chiropractor, they only initiated the referral approximately 11.5% of the time and preferred that patients contact the chiropractor on their own. The authors discuss later in the study that this may be indicative of an unwillingness to formalize their relationships with chiropractors, the fear of malpractice litigation, or perhaps the fear of competition.

If a Doctor Exhibits One of These Concerns, How Should You Handle It?

In regard to competition, medical doctors should not fear competition. Chiropractors compete over where doctors send their patients for back pain treatments; we do not take their patients from them. Be sure when asking for referrals that you clarify that you will not only keep the doctor in the loop regarding patient progress but also that the patient will remain the doctor's patient.

Regarding formalizing the relationship with chiropractors, consumer demand is pushing doctors to form relationships with alternative care providers. Why can't this alternative care provider be a chiropractor?

Regarding the fear of litigation, a study published in *Annals of Internal Medicine* by Cohen and Eisenberg outlines concerns and trends that lead to concern by medical physicians when referring patients for alternative care.[3] The bottom line is that doctors can be liable for negligently prescribing "unsafe" care. Alternative care that doesn't have a known risk or in which the risk is very small would be recommended. Alternative care such as nutritional supplementation that may cause a known drug-to-drug interaction would probably not be recommended. For chiropractic care, safety is most likely a concern as far as liability is concerned. This is easily overcome by presenting the research documenting not only efficacy but safety as well. Also related to the issue of safety when referring to chiropractors is that doctors don't understand that chiropractors know how to differentially diagnose or that we are educated on how to watch for signs of serious adverse reactions. You can easily explain this using research and discussing the chiropractic education and history and physical process.

Providing Case Reports

On average allopathic care providers "usually and always provide a case report with referral" 66% of the time. However, when referring a patient to a chiropractor, this number crashes to just over 10%. The numbers are similar for sending X-rays: 63% to an allopathic provider and just under 10% for a chiropractor. In my opinion, this doesn't support the notion of a true referral, but rather a referral that was either lumped together with a referral to a massage therapist or acupuncturist or one suggested by the patient in which the doctor simply said yes.

Another question in the study asked how often allopathic providers included a reason for the referral.[2] When referring to each other, the rate was 91%. However, when asked if allopathic providers provided a reason for referral to chiropractors, the result indicated they did so only 17% of the time. In contrast, doctors in this study reported that they may not accept a referral from a chiropractor because of the absence of a formal referral. Eighteen percent of DOs and 19% of MDs indicated that chiropractors did not send them any clinical information. When it came to a report of findings, 62% of physicians routinely provided a report of findings to another medical doctor but provided the report of findings only 25% of the time to a chiropractor.[2]

These are important findings. Doctors feel that chiropractors should report to them but do not feel that they need to report to chiropractors. Doctors don't view chiropractors as equals, and their lack in providing any diagnostic information or clinical history means they may not understand that this provides as much information to chiropractors as it does to medical doctors. These findings illustrate that medical doctors do not understand the scientific component and educational background of the chiropractic industry. As part of a provider service, it is a professional courtesy to both the patient and the attending doctor that a reason for referral and brief case history be provided to ensure continuity of care.

Oftentimes chiropractors turn to their patients to see what the follow-up with the medical doctor was. This is not only detrimental to proper patient care, but it also serves to accentuate in the patient's mind the gap that continues to exist between medical and chiropractic physicians, not to mention possibly undermining patient confidence.

Characteristics of Doctors Most Likely to Respond Favorably to a Chiropractor

Greene et al. mention that one of the greatest driving forces for the PCP to refer or recommend to chiropractors is the patient's own interest.[2] In addition, studies have found that providers refer their patients for alternative care primarily for a musculoskeletal condition. This was consistent with the Greene et al. findings that the most frequent reason for referral to a chiropractor was *"chronic musculoskeletal pain that does not respond to conventional treatments."*[2]

The doctors most likely to show a positive referral attitude toward chiropractors were the following:

- A PCP in private practice.
- Younger physicians.
- Female physicians are more open to view complementary and alternative medicine as useful.
- Male physicians are more likely to have accepted referrals from chiropractors.

Communication Issues

Finally, Greene et al. note that the source of poor interprofessional chiropractic and medical relations is related to poor communications and a negative attitude by PCPs in Iowa toward chiropractors. Can you imagine the possibilities achievable simply by utilizing a professional approach and educating doctors on the research and safety of manipulation? In doing so, you can illustrate that you are a responsible and ethical healthcare provider.

The next study illustrates how physicians like to be communicated with as well as their thoughts on some of our terminology.

"Communication Between General Practitioners and Chiropractors." William J. Brussee, Willem J. J. Assendelft, and Alan C. Breen. *Journal of Manipulative and Physiological Therapeutics.* 2001;24:12–16.

Abstract

Objective: Good communication between health care professionals has proved to be important in ensuring high standards of care. Patients have shown an increased use of complementary medicine (eg, chiropractic) in addition to conventional medicine.

However, this does not automatically guarantee good cooperation and communication between complementary practitioners and conventional practitioners. The objective of this study was to assess the nature and quality of communication between general practitioners and chiropractors (in The Netherlands) and to look for areas for improvement.

Design and Setting: Postal questionnaires were sent to general practitioners requesting personal and practice details and asking about their knowledge of chiropractic, present communications, opinions on chiropractic terminology, and preferences with regard to communications with patients.

Subjects: A total of 252 general practitioners in 84 Dutch cities.

Results: A total of 115 questionnaires (46%) were returned. Almost all of the general practitioners had at least heard of chiropractic. Most information came from patients who were treated by chiropractors (78%). Only 10% of the general practitioners refer their patients to a chiropractor on a regular basis. Referral of patients was found to be significantly related to the general practitioners' perceived knowledge of chiropractic and positive opinions regarding their past communications with chiropractors. More than 80% of the general practitioners said that they were interested in receiving (or continuing to receive) feedback reports, even if they did not personally refer the patient to the chiropractor. Chiropractic feedback reports often seem to contain confusing terminology (40%), which might negatively influence communication (66%). General practitioners preferred a typed (88%), short (69%) feedback report, preferably sent after the last treatment (72%).

Conclusions: The results of this study show most general practitioners to have a neutral to positive attitude toward communication with chiropractors. The general practitioners' preferences with regard to the technical aspects of a feedback report concur with the results of similar surveys in the field and can be used as guidelines for written communications. Factors that negatively influence communication between general practitioners and chiropractors seem to be confusing terminology, a limited knowledge of chiropractic, and bad experiences in previous communications. Recognition and illumination of these factors are a prerequisite to the development of good communication.

This study[4] is very illuminating. We know there are communication issues between chiropractors and allopathic doctors. Part of the chiropractic college curriculum discusses the difference between a chiropractic subluxation and a medical subluxation. If we are to promote to medical doctors, we need to learn what language to speak to maximize our efforts and what words we might say and the way in which to communicate (verbal or written) that will aid us in our promotional efforts and bridge the gap between the two professions.

As you promote to physicians, understand that the manner in which you approach them (verbal or by letter) and the words that you utilize in the process affect the relationship. Realize that you can cause alienation by using some "chiropractic"-specific words.[4] Points to remember from this study are the following:

- "A statistically significant relationship was found between the level of knowledge of chiropractic and the frequency of referral of patients to a chiropractor."[4]
- Doctors prefer to receive information about chiropractic through presentations, scientific literature, and correspondence with chiropractors about patients.[4] With this text, you have the tools and literature with which to do this with confidence.
- The evidence exists for chiropractors to confidently assume their rightful place in the healthcare arena, especially in the treatment of lower back, neck, and headaches.

- Referrals won't come directly to you unless you have and provide good communication with medical doctors. This means not only in promotions but in patient report of findings as well.

- The approach chiropractors take in treating patients is contradictory to medical doctors. This, in combination with academic backgrounds and professional jargon, can lead to professional misunderstandings and poor professional relationships.

- Ten percent of MDs refer patients to chiropractors; of this 10%, 35% did not make referrals often and another 35% only made referrals at the patient's request.[4]

- "A statistically significant relationship was found between a positive opinion of previous communications and the frequency of referring patient to chiropractors."[4]

- When asked about typed reports, the MDs' preferences were as follows:
  - One report at the end of treatment.
  - Length of report to be between one-half and 1 full page.
  - Omit findings and terminology that a doctor wouldn't understand. For instance, avoid words that can be confusing such as *kinematic, level of compensation, myofascial trigger point, discogenic,* and *entrapment.* Appendix J provides a sample report.
  - When you begin a referral relationship with an MD, you can clarify which report pattern he or she prefers. You might also include one in your detail binder.

- When asked about information they would like to hear about, "The primary response was to find out the treatment indications and the difference between manual therapy and chiropractic."

- Some stereotypes were also elicited in the comments section and have already been addressed in this text:
  - Maintenance care (Concerns can be defeated utilizing any of the studies on efficacy because they illustrate short treatment durations and reasonable treatment frequency.)
  - Financial (Concerns can be defeated not only with cost-efficacy data but with your explanation of the services you provide. Hint: Don't try to sell a doctor on the virtues of maintenance care. The evidence isn't supportive and is in fact contradictory to the positive efficacy studies.)

In summary, there is little room to doubt that consumers are demanding chiropractic care and allopathic care providers are recommending it. They just won't recommend a specific chiropractic doctor. Imagine the potential referral business you can gain simply by illustrating to MDs the benefits of chiropractic care and which patients would be appropriate to refer. Doctors' attitudes may switch from one of "yes, you could see someone like a chiropractor or massage therapist" to "A chiropractor can benefit your condition. I am comfortable referring you to Dr. Acampora because I know her treatment protocol and examination process." In addition, we now understand doctors' dislike of chiropractic terms, so stick with the talk the researchers talk. Doctors don't care what segment you are adjusting or in what direction the spinous process is pointing; they just want to know what we do. If we want their business, we need to educate them through research. Doing so will make a tremendous impact on bridging the gap between the two professions.

What Do the Guidelines Currently Advocate for Back Pain from a PCP Point of View?

The papers presented in this section are meant only to acquaint you with current common guidelines for the treatment of lower back pain. They illustrate how a doctor approaches back pain, the treatment protocols available, and the recommendations and reviews of these available treatments. Let's start with the most recent:

"Diagnosis and Treatment of Low Back Pain: A Joint Clinical Practice Guidelines from the American College of Physicians and the American Pain Society." Roger Chou, Amir Qaseem, Vincenza Snow, Donald Casey, J. Thomas Cross Jr., Paul Shekelle, and Douglas K. Owens, for the Clinical Efficacy Assessment Subcommittee of the American College of Physicians and the American College of Physicians/ American Pain Society Low Back Pain Guidelines Panel. *Annals of Internal Medicine.* October 2007.

The recommendation focused on spinal manipulation is as follows:

> Recommendation 7: For patients who do not improve with self-care options, clinicians should consider the addition of nonpharmacologic therapy with proven benefits—for acute low back pain, spinal

manipulation; for chronic or subacute low back pain, intensive interdisciplinary rehabilitation, exercise therapy, acupuncture, massage therapy, spinal manipulation, yoga, cognitive-behavioral therapy, or progressive relaxation (weak recommendation, moderate-quality evidence).[5]

and

The evidence is insufficient to conclude that benefits of manipulation vary according to the profession of the manipulator (chiropractor vs. other clinician trained in manipulation) or according to presence or absence of radiating pain.[6]

Unfortunately, this review, though stating that it performed MedLine medical searches from 1966 through November 2006, cites only a few important chiropractic research papers despite several that were also available during the time of the search parameters.[5]

Of the studies they did cite, the first study was conducted in 1998 by Dr. Cherkin and associates and compared physical therapy, manipulation, and provision of an educational booklet. The conclusions were that physical therapy and manipulation were similar in cost and effect.[7] The second study cited is the 1994 Agency for Health Care Policy and Research (AHCPR) Clinical Practice Guideline discussed further in this chapter.[8] The third study cited is a meta-analysis by Dr. Assendelft and colleagues completed in 2003.[6] The paper received some criticism because the studies included in the analysis were not homogenous in nature and the effect of manipulation was not always clear. The fourth study cited is a paper published in 2004 in the *Annals of Internal Medicine* that used a clinical prediction rule to identify patients most likely to respond to spinal manipulation; manipulation was performed by physical therapists.[9]

The intention of the Chou et al. paper is to illustrate treatment options for lower back pain. Unfortunately, many qualified evidence-based chiropractic research findings were not included. It is an incomplete assessment that fails to differentiate many important components of treatments, including the specific type of back pain, the duration of the back pain, the effect of treatment on pain and disability, the cost of treatments, and the trend of consumer demand for alternative health care. The evidence that exists for manipulation is enough to command its own recommendation similar to the attention the authors paid to medication. There is simply too much information on manipulation to try to summarize it in a group of treatments that don't have the same level of available research. On a positive note, at least the article mentions spinal manipulation as a treatment option.

"Spinal Manipulation." *The Medical Letter on Drugs and Therapeutics.* 2002;44 (1132).

The *Medical Letter on Drugs and Therapeutics* seems to specialize in finding the one worst research article and then reporting it despite the overwhelming positive and contradictory research. The following is the *Medical Letter's* conclusion regarding manipulation:

> CONCLUSION—Spinal manipulation can cause life-threatening complications. Manipulation of the cervical spine, which has been associated with dissection of the vertebral artery, appears to be especially dangerous.[10]

This conclusion is based in part on commentaries, not scientific papers, two of which are the product of a researcher who seems to be very biased against the chiropractic profession. That such a strong warning is associated with manipulation when most papers are unable to provide a direct link to danger is biased and inflammatory. In addition, the paper focuses on the unusual treatment indications for which manipulation was not proven to be efficacious such as asthma, enuresis, and dysmenorrhea, while ignoring the overwhelming positive findings for lower back pain. My experience leads me to place little value in *Medical Letter* conclusions, but you may hear about this publication in doctors' offices. This particular article is outdated, and enough research has been published to refute this ill-supported "conclusion."

"Evaluation and Treatment of Acute Low Back Pain." Scott Kincade. *American Family Physician.* 2007;75(8):1181–1188.

Although not a research article or formal government treatment guideline, this does offer the family physician an overview of the diagnosis and treatment options for lower back pain.

Page 1182 of the study provides a table of "clinical recommendations" with an evidence rating for the different choices.[11] Although it is a recent publication, it did not include the recent NSAID warning from the American Heart Association. Figure 5–1 is adapted from this study.

Cochrane Back Group

The Cochrane Database is well known by physicians and is a common reference site for treatment reviews.[12]

Evidence Rating

1. 4 to 6 weeks of conservative care for acute lower back   C
   pain without absence of red flags
2. NSAID, acetaminophen, and muscle relaxants   A
6. Heat therapy may help reduce pain and increase function   B
7. "Spinal manipulation therapy for acute low back pain   B
   may offer short-term benefits but probably is no more
   effective than usual medical care"

A = consistent, good-quality patient-oriented evidence; B = inconsistent or limited-quality patient-oriented evidence; C = consensus, disease-oriented evidence, usual practice, expert opinion, or case series. For information about the SORT evidence rating system, see page 1135 of the study or http://www.aafp.org/afpsort.xml.

Source: Kinkade S. Evaluation and treatment of acute low back pain. *Am Fam Phys.* 2007; 75:1181-1188,1190-1192.

Figure 5–1   *Clinical recommendations and associated evidence ratings for acute lower back pain.*

The Cochrane Group concludes the following for manipulation and low back pain:

> There was little or no difference in pain reduction or the ability to perform everyday activities between people with low-back pain who received spinal manipulation and those who received other advocated therapies.

"Spinal Manipulative Therapy for Low-Back Pain." Assendelft WJJ, Morton SC, YU Emily I, Suttorp MJ, Shekelle PG. Cochrane Database of Systematic Reviews 2004. Issue 1. Art No: CO 000447. DOI:10. 1002/14651858. CD000447. pub 2. (www.cochrane.org/reviews/en/ab000447.html)

As we will see in Chapter 8, "The Evidence for Efficacy of Manipulation," a systematic review by Bronfort et al. in 2004 improved on the methodology for which studies were included in the review and this study could be used to overcome the Assendelft study that had the following conclusions.

For neck pain:

> People with neck pain, as well as people with neck pain plus related headache that lasted at least one month, who received

multimodal care that included exercises plus mobilization (movement imposed onto joints and muscles) or manipulation (adjustments) reported greater pain reduction, improved ability to perform everyday activities and an increase in their perceived effects of treatment than those who received no treatment."

Cervical Overview Group. "Manipulation and Mobilisation for Mechanical Neck Disorders." Gross AR, Hoving JL, Hains TA, et al. Cochrane Database of Systematic Reviews. 2004, Issue 1. Art No: CD004249.DOI: 10.1002/14651858.CD004249. pub 2. (www.cochrane.org/reviews/en/ab004249.html)

Agency for Health Care Policy and Research

Acute Low Back Pain Problems in Adults: Assessment and Treatment. S. Bigos, O. Bowyer, G. Braen, et al. Quick Reference Guide for Clinicians. Clinical Practice Guideline No. 14. Rockville, MD: Agency for Health Care Policy and Research; 1994.

Because of the year of publication and the large amount of new research validating chiropractic manipulation in all major categories (efficacy, safety, cost, and patient satisfaction), this guideline is outdated.[7] In addition, this report is limited only to acute low back pain. Manipulation can be found under the heading "Physical Methods." Specifically, the article states:

> Manipulation, defined as manual loading of the spine using short or long leverage methods, is safe and effective for patients in the first month of acute low back symptoms without radiculopathy. For patients with symptoms lasting longer than 1 month, manipulation is probably safe but its efficacy is unproven. If manipulation has not resulted in symptomatic and functional improvement after 4 weeks, it should be stopped and the patient reevaluated."[7]

Chapter 8, "The Evidence for Efficacy of Manipulation," in this book covers new research that proves efficacy of manipulation for chronic and acute lower back pain. There have not been any new updates to these clinical practice guidelines. As the title of this article states, this was one of several clinical guidelines for a variety of conditions.

Another AHCPR review of manipulation can be found on the AHCPR Web site and is also available through ChiroWeb.

"Benefits and Risks of Spinal Manipulation." Paul G. Shekelle, Reed B. Phillips, Daniel C. Cherkin, William C. Meeker. In: Cherkin DC, Mootz RD, eds. *Chiropractic in the United States: Training, Practice, and Research.* AHCPR Publication No. 98-N002. Rockville, MD: Agency for Health Care Policy and Research; 1997.

As the title suggests, this report outlines all the information available on manipulation. The most recent study cited in the references was published in 1997, so this article is outdated, too.[13] The overall impression of this review is similar to others of its time in that efficacy research is not consistent and that there is limited quality research from which to draw conclusions. Regarding safety, the review covers a fair assessment of benign side effects and documents that a rare risk for more serious side effects exists. Patient satisfaction was noted to be consistent, and the cost-effectiveness data were not properly controlled in trials. Since this time, as you will see in the upcoming chapters, many new high-quality studies are available for all of these categories.

The Most Common Objections to Expect

Chiropractors do not treat and release:

1. The number one expected objection for medical doctors will most likely be: "The problem with chiropractors is that patients have to keep going back." Without a doubt, many chiropractors have promoted this philosophy. The problem is there is no evidence-based research to substantiate the benefit to the patient of such maintenance care. As such, doctors are leery of referring their patients for chiropractic care. In the efficacy sections of the research articles, all of the studies illustrate a modest frequency and duration of treatment. Emphasize this in your presentations and practice it. Obviously, not all patients follow the research. Some patients may need more care, but usually such patients have coexisting conditions, his-

tory of multiple back injuries, or another reason requiring the need for more than the usual care.

Cervical manipulation and safety:

2. When promoting cervical manipulation, the number one concern for a doctor is safety. "I don't mind if you treat lower backs, but I won't refer a cervical pain patient because of risk of stroke." The safety of manipulation is discussed in-depth in Chapter 9, and many research papers are provided with which you can overcome this objection.

Treating outside scope of care:

3. Another popular objection is: "Chiropractors think they can treat any condition." Again, relying on the evidence to promote chiropractors as specialists of neuromuscular conditions will add to your credibility. Providing the doctor with conditions that are contraindicated for chiropractic care as well as providing a list of common conditions that are indicated for chiropractic care can help satisfy this objection.

Financial:

4. Another objection will likely be centered on financial concerns. This will take some clarifying. Is the doctor concerned about managed care overtreating or concerned that you will be selling nutritional supplementations to every patient?

   In the case of managed care, provide the most common insurance companies that you accept will help to alleviate that concern.

   In the case of providing nutritional supplementation, you will have to overcome the objection when it is announced. It has already been mentioned that nutritional supplements cause concern for doctors because of drug-to-drug interactions and their lack of regulation by the Food and Drug Administration. The bottom line here is again to resort to the evidence and to follow the guidelines. A diagnosis of lower back pain does not imply the necessity of nutritional supplementation. The patients in the studies were not made better by supplementation; they were made better by manipulation.

   Overtreating was discussed earlier, but again rely on the evidence to validate the cost of care with eight or so treatments.

The next few chapters explore the research and how it can be successfully communicated to the medical community.

REFERENCES

1. Antman EM, Bennett JS, Daugherty A, Furberg C, Roberts H, Taubert KA. Use of nonsteroidal anti-inflammatory drugs. An update for clinicians. A scientific statement from the American Heart Association. *Circulation.* 2007;115(12):1634–1642.

2. Greene B, Smith M, Allareddy V, Haas M. Referral patterns and attitudes of primary care physicians towards chiropractors. *BMC Complementary Alternative Med.* 2006;6:5.

3. Cohen M, Eisenberg D. Potential physician malpractice liability associated with complementary and integrative medical therapies. *Ann Intern Med.* 2002;136:596–603.

4. Brussee W, Assendelft W, Breen A. Communication between general practitioners and chiropractors. *J Manipulative Physiol Ther.* 2001;24:12–16.

5. Chou R, Qaseem A, Snow V, et al., for the Clinical Efficacy Assessment Subcommittee of the American College of Physicians and the American College of Physicians/American Pain Society Low Back Pain Guidelines Panel. Diagnosis and treatment of low back pain: a joint clinical practice guideline from the American College of Physicians and the American Pain Society. *Ann Intern Med.* October 2007;147:478–491.

6. Assendelft WJ, Morton SC, Yu EI, Suttorp MJ, Shekelle PG. Spinal manipulative therapy for low back pain. A meta-analysis of effectiveness relative to other therapies. *Ann Intern Med.* 2003;138:871–881.

7. Cherkin DC, Deyo RA, Battié M, Street J, Barlow W. A comparison of physical therapy, chiropractic manipulation, and provision of an educational booklet for the treatment of patients with low back pain. *N Engl J Med.* 1998;339(15):1021–1029.

8. Bigos S, Bowyer O, Braen G, et al. *Acute Low Back Problems in Adults.* Clinical Practice Guideline No. 14. AHCPR Publication No. 95-0642. Rockville, MD: Agency for Health Care Policy and Research, Public Health Service, US Department of Health and Human Services; 1994.

9. Childs M, Fritz J, Flynn T, et al. A clinical prediction rule to identify patients with low back pain most likely to benefit from spinal manipulation: a validation study. *Ann Intern Med.* 2004;141:920–928.

10. The Medical Letter on Drugs and Therapeutics. Spinal manipulation. *Med Lett Drugs Ther.* 2002;44:1132.

11. Kincade S. Evaluation and treatment of low back pain. *Am Fam Phys.* 2007;75(8): 1181–1188.

12. French SD, Grant WE, Green S, Walker B. Chiropractic interventions for low-back pain (protocol). *Cochrane Database of Systematic Reviews.* 2005;(3):art. no. CD005427.

13. Shekelle PG, Phillips RB, Cherkin DC, Meeker WC. Benefits and risks of spinal manipulation. In: Cherkin DC, Mootz RD, eds. *Chiropractic in the United States: Training, Practice, and Research.* AHCPR Publication No. 98-N002. Rockville, MD: Agency for Health Care Policy and Research, 1997.

Chapter 6

Research and Evidence-Based Chiropractic

Unreasonable leaps of faith and dogma inhibit understanding of the physiological effects of the adjustment and slows down eventual comprehension of the value of chiropractic care.
—Scott Haldeman, DC, "Evolution of Chiropractic—Science and Research"

I t is difficult to dedicate enough time to review the ever-growing body of evidence-based chiropractic research. Yet, in today's ever-changing health environment it is impossible to integrate with medicine and managed care and not be up-to-date on key research and evidence-based chiropractic. Abstracts and professional summaries on key research highlight the existence of research studies and what the studies focus on, but they cannot provide a thorough understanding of the findings and conclusions. Certainly, medical doctors have embraced the evidence-based healthcare movement and frequently cite findings in studies to justify their treatment recommendations to their patients. To remain an integral player in health care, chiropractors need to follow the trend.

In conjunction with this trend, many books on evidence-based health care have been published. One text that I refer to frequently throughout this section and the subsequent chapters dedicated to understanding research is *Evidence-Based Chiropractic Practice* by Michael Haneline.[1] This essential book informs readers about the procedures involved in the practice of evidence-based chiropractic care and provides background information that is necessary for obtaining and interpreting chiropractic evidence, as well as practical examples to assist with implementation. The book also offers important information on understanding the content of research articles, including the basics of research design and biostatistics—information that is vital to rendering optimal patient care.

David Sackett, who helped identify and create evidence-based practice, defines evidence-based medicine as follows: "Evidence-based medicine is the conscientious, explicit, and judicious use of current best evidence in making decisions about the care of individual patients. The practice of evidence-based medicine means integrating individual clinical expertise with the best available external clinical evidence from systematic research."[2]

With the availability of the Internet and the initiative of many consumers who are willing to research their own conditions that drive the consumer-driven managed care arena, chiropractic doctors must now more than ever practice treatments that have been proven to be effective. This is not to say that clinical experience no longer counts for anything. In fact, it does, but it is a balance between clinical experience and the most current research that allows us to provide the best care for our patients.

Managed care mirrors this expectation, albeit in a darker setting, through the changing and diminished reimbursements. Provider report cards are now being examined, and your treatment plan is compared against the general population. Knowing how to use evidence-based research to receive reimbursement is becoming routine in most chiropractic practices.

As you will see in some of the research studies, conclusions are drawn based on insurance statistics using Current Procedural Terminology and International Classification of Diseases data. These data are pooled together to draw conclusions on the efficacy of manipulation, length of treatment, diagnostic procedures, patient demographics, and more. Managed care, from a provider perspective, isn't only about reimbursements anymore.

Research is not always the most tantalizing reading; however, from a promotional perspective it can get pretty close. In medical sales, your presentation is only as good as your research. For chiropractors trying to break into the medical world, there is nothing better than research that proves efficacy through treatment of the spine. In this discussion of research from a promotional perspective, you will learn how to use research to educate doctors on the benefits of our services. Manipulation has gained some notoriety in the treatment of the spine. With baby boomers demanding a more holistic and affordable healthcare approach, doctors are ready to listen.

Research Resources

Research is ever changing and there is always a major research project under way. Although there are several resources available on the Internet, the ones that stand out as good to consult for current updates on research and evidenced-based chiropractic are these:

Foundation for Chiropractic Education and Research (FCER)
   (http://www.FCER.org)

Palmer Center for Chiropractic Research
   (http://www.palmer.edu/research.aspx)

Council on Chiropractic Guidelines and Practice Parameters
   (http://www.ccgpp.org)

National Center for Complementary and Alternative Medicine (NCCAM)
   (http://nccam.nih.gov)

These Web sites are tremendous sources of information for research and evidence-based health care. I encourage you to visit the Web sites, and I especially encourage you to support chiropractic research by becoming a member of the FCER.

Today chiropractic manipulation enjoys strong and compelling evidence for the treatment of the lower back, neck, and some types of headaches. Chiropractic's professional research is continuing to evolve into other areas, and we can hope that in the next few years data will be published that can be used to illustrate chiropractic efficacy for other conditions. Some research has proved manipulation to be ineffective. We must be willing to accept the bad with the good. No research paper is void of any negative findings, and you should expect to see this even in the clinicals that you promote to physicians. If the *overall* theme of the paper is positive and the study design is sound, you have something that you can promote and that will hold up over time until a new and updated study takes its place.

As you gain physicians' trust and professional respect, you will be able to promote other conditions that chiropractors are qualified to treat, provided that you have properly educated a doctor on the science that explains manipulation as well as the science that proves its efficacy and safety. Assuming that you did this well and have received patient referrals, you will want to make sure that you provide those patients with competent, reasonable care and that the doctor knows the results his or her patients achieved while in your care. Once the doctor trusts you to make sound clinical judgments and understands the type of care you provide, his or her mind will be open to extending that care to other neuromuscular disorders such as carpal tunnel syndrome, ankle sprains, and so on. Until that time comes, stick to promoting the most common complaints that chiropractors treat, which are supported by a profound body of evidence.

A problem chiropractic practitioners face with staying current on research is the exorbitant cost to do so, especially for those journals that have annual fees of $500 or more. Several options are available to chiropractors to limit these costs. Aligned Methods (http://www.alignedmethods.com) is one option for chiropractors who wish to stay current with research that can be used in a promotional setting. For a nominal monthly fee, Aligned Methods provides frequent e-mail updates as new research is released both for chiropractic and its competitors in scientific journals. Aligned Methods also provides public relations event ideas and continues to enhance the promotional efforts between MDs, DOs, and chiropractors by providing promotional techniques and ideas.

Another option for those who are fortunate enough to live by a chiropractic college, is to take advantage of the full and free access to most journal articles the library provides. A quarterly visit to the library for a few hours should provide you with the major scientific updates, which you can then print and read when you have time. If you don't live by a college, your options are more limited. Many scientific journals allow you to set up an online request for e-mail notification when a new issue is released. These journals will then e-mail you the monthly table of contents, and if a title in the table of contents is of interest, you can usually purchase it individually.

In addition to the journals, Pub Med (free) and Manual Alternative and Natural Therapy Index Systems (MANTIS; subscription cost) are online search engines that allow you to set up searches that alert you via e-mail about new content as it is posted that meets your search criteria. One final option is to become a member of the American Chiropractic Association (ACA) and the FCER. A membership with the ACA provides free access to the *Journal of Manipulative and Physiological Therapeutics,* and the FCER membership provides you with free access to MANTIS.

Literature Searches

There are several search engines available. It is easiest to pick one or two such as PubMed and MANTIS. PubMed is a well-known search engine for medical doctors with the added perk of providing free searches. MANTIS is available as part of FCER membership benefits. Advanced search techniques can find relevant literature fast. Dr. Michael Haneline's text provides an in-depth discussion on literature searches.[1] He describes several search engines available on the Internet, including the two listed here, for which the following descriptions are provided:

PubMed

PubMed includes over 15 million (and growing) citations for biomedical articles dating back to the 1950s. These citations are from MEDLINE and additional life science journals. MEDLINE itself has nearly 13 million records from 1966 to the present. PubMed includes links to many sites providing full-text articles and other related resources. PubMed is a service of the National Library of Medicine. URL: http://PubMed.gov

CAM on PubMed: CAM on PubMed is a subset of the PubMed database that was created through a partnership between the National Center for Complementary and Alternative Medicine and the National Library of Medicine. CAM on PubMed uses a feature to locate citations with a predetermined CAM search criterion. This feature can be utilized directly from PubMed by choosing "Limits" and "Complementary Medicine" from the Subsets menu. Currently there are over 270,000 citations in the CAM subset of PubMed from 1966 forward. URL: http://www.nlm.nih.gov/nccam/camonpubmed.html[1]

MANTIS

Manual Alternative and Natural Therapy Index System (MANTIS): MANTIS addresses all areas of alternative medical literature. It covers health care disciplines not significantly represented in the major biomedical databases and includes references from more than 1,400 journals, with preference given to peer-reviewed journals. MANTIS began including the full text of alternative medical journals in the fall of 1999. Produced by Action Potential, it has become the largest index of peer-reviewed journals for several disciplines, including chiropractic, osteopathy, homeopathy, and manual medicine. URL: http://www.healthindex.com[1]

There is one final option for information to which chiropractors can subscribe. More than likely, you may hear about this from the medical profession. For a fee, the Cochrane Library provides a collection of evidence for specific conditions such as lower back pain. A brief description as listed in Dr. Haneline's book is provided:

The Cochrane Library

Consists of eight regularly updated evidence-based databases, all of which are concerned with the effects of interventions in health care. The Cochrane Library is designed to provide information and evidence to support decisions taken in health care and to inform those receiving care. The Cochrane database of systematic reviews is full text, whereas most of the other databases contain primarily citations and abstracts. Published on a quarterly basis. URL: http://www.thecochranelibrary.org[1]

These and other search engines allow you to set up alerts that will notify you when new publications or articles that meet your criteria are published. Searching on these sites is fairly straightforward, and the more searches you perform, the more accustomed you will become to using these tools.

Determining Credibility of a Journal Article for Promotional Purposes

For the chiropractic promotional process, the information you bring a doctor relating to manipulation must be strong and the doctor must be able to identify with the proof source. The following factors are important to doctors:

1. Journal publication
2. Date of publication (some exceptions apply)
3. Author credentials
4. Methodology
5. Study participants (the n)
6. Objective measurements
7. The p value (statistical significance)
8. Conclusions

The Journal Publication

When you introduce a study from which you are citing data, in one of the first sentences you should provide the name of the journal in which the research is published as well as the date of publication. Failing to validate the data source and diving into the research can result in the doctor missing the data while searching for the publication information. Introducing research can begin with something similar to: "Doctor, in the November 2007 issue of the *Journal of Manipulative and Physiological Therapeutics . . .*"

The journal from which you pull your research should be included on Index Medicus because a listing on Index Medicus has built-in credibility and limits any objection a doctor can have on where the data come from. Index Medicus is a listing of worldwide publications of medical literature, which has been deemed to be most useful by a group of medical physicians, editors, and librarians. The National Library of Medicine and the National Institute of Health provide a search of these publications through PubMed. The *Journal of Manipulative and Physiological Therapeutics (JMPT)* is included in Index Medicus. If you provide the doctor with a publication not listed on Index Medicus, the credibility of your research article may diminish. This is not to imply that the publication produces bad research; it is noted from a promotional standpoint. You want to have the doctor provide objections that can be overcome by solid research; you don't want to start off the promotional effort justifying the journal. For chiropractic publications, the main journal that meets these criteria is the *JMPT*. Most likely, the doctor may not know of *JMPT*, so you will need to be able to explain the following facts about *JMPT* to doctors:

- Is included on Index Medicus (this adds instant credibility).
- Is peer reviewed.
- Has an editorial board consisting of notable clinical researchers from the chiropractic, medical, and osteopathic fields.
- Readers include chiropractors, osteopaths, physical therapists, psychiatrists, radiologists, and sports medicine specialists.
- Provides the latest information on current developments in therapeutics, as well as reviews of clinically oriented research and practical information for use in clinical settings.

JMPT is an outstanding journal and will certainly be a source of much of the literature you present to physicians. Despite this, you may find a doctor who objects, saying that *JMPT* is biased simply because it is a product of the chiropractic profession. Although this is an unwarranted objection, because *JMPT* is peer reviewed by medical professionals outside of the chiropractic industry, you might as well cite data from other journal publications. It is difficult to overcome this type of bias objection, and other journals provide promotional material for chiropractors, too. This is usually a rare objection to *JMPT*. Once you gain rapport and professional trust, you can revisit *JMPT*.

Articles published in such magazines as *Sports Illustrated* or *Ladies Home Journal* are not research articles and are not appropriate for promotional efforts. Likewise, a doctor who hears of some piece of negative literature in such a magazine should know that the source is not reputable for scientific purposes. Beware that articles in popular magazines are usually sensationalized and based on a few isolated cases and lack scientific credibility.

Publication Date

For the most part, utilize research that is recent. Using evidence in favor of manipulation compared to some other therapy that is now obsolete won't exactly sell the doctor on manipulation. Defining *recent* can be tricky. For example, the data I cite in this text were primarily published in 2000 and later, with the majority published in the past 5 years. The only reason you would use research published earlier than 5 years ago is because the research in its entirety is still standard treatment in today's healthcare environment options *and* no updated research has been published. That said, this is one more reason to stay current on research. Research that replaces the research cited in this text will be noted on the Aligned Methods Web site and through membership alerts. You can perform searches for new data and interpret the evidence on your own as well.

Author Credentials

This is straightforward. Studies done solely by doctors of chiropractic may be perceived as potentially biased, especially from a safety perspective. If you start with a study for which all authors are chiropractors and the doctor objects to the data based on bias, you can try to overcome the objection by clarifying the validity of the study design and methodology, or you can cite a different study where authors are a mix of healthcare professionals. If you get this objection, you should assume there is a mistrust of "chiropractic" research for whatever reason. However, the doctor has allowed you to get this far, so clearly he or she is interested in learning more about chiropractic services and manipulation. As you gain credibility, you will most likely be able to move back to citing chiropractic research.

Methodology

In the simplest terms, methodology describes why and how the study authors completed the research project. The many components of a study discussed in the Methods section of a report are beyond the scope of this book, but some pertinent highlights are discussed here. Also, Dr. Haneline's book[1] can provide a more detailed explanation.

Study Design

Study design can usually be described in two or three words as you present your data. The following are the most common:

Randomized controlled study This is the most popular of all research study designs because it is the most effective at removing any bias. *Bias* is not always intentional in the sense that the authors created a study design that perpetuates the findings they wanted to see. Bias can also occur unintentionally at several points in the study. If you introduce a study that is a *double blind* (neither the patients nor the doctors knew which treatment was being administered) *randomized controlled study,* the results are most likely related to the treatment that was administered, with almost no bias to interfere with the results. In the pharmaceutical world, this is the main type of study doctors expect to see because it is easy to blind both the patients and the doctors to the treatment. However, in the chiropractic world, how do you blind a doctor from knowing whether he or she delivered an adjustment? How do you blind the patient? Patients might still be able to tell the difference between a sham procedure and a real adjustment. Double-blind studies are extremely difficult to produce for physical medicines such as manipulation, and if blinding is noted in the study design, usually the person who gathers the information was blinded. Single-blind studies have been conducted with more success. *Randomization* means that the control group and the treatment group have a similar characteristic makeup or patient demographic. For instance, if you averaged each group's pain level, the averages would be fairly similar. Randomization in many studies doesn't necessarily mean that a *placebo treatment or control group* was utilized. It might mean three different treatments were used, and the choice depends largely on the objective of the study. In the UK BEAM trial, a study that is examined in the next few chapters, the authors sought to determine from a general practitioner standpoint what effect on back pain would occur by adding to their standard care one of three different treatments:

1. Physical therapy
2. Manipulation
3. Combination of physical therapy and manipulation

For the UK BEAM trial, the control group was the patients who had general practitioner care only.

Pragmatic Study A pragmatic study closely mirrors a physician's practice and determines how one treatment works compared to other treatments. For promotional purposes, these are useful studies because they relate to what the doctor can expect to see in his own office, or better yet the outcomes the doctor will likely see in his patients.

Meta-analysis (systematic reviews) A meta-analysis review combines several studies into one study; however, it is important that the studies being combined are homogenous. From a promotional perspective, a meta-analysis study is helpful because it combines several studies and data together, creating a larger patient base, which adds to the validity of the study and makes the findings more meaningful. The problem with meta-analyses is that different authors can reach different conclusions after analyzing the same data.

This description of study designs is not all inclusive but most likely covers the types of designs you will see most frequently in research.

The Methods section of a study is the place to consult for all the study specifics. For instance, how did the researchers pick the patients and how did they randomize them? What were the inclusion/exclusion criteria? What software did the researchers use for statistical pooling and so on? Essentially, the Methods section gives you every detail that you would need to recreate the study and reproduce the results. Most doctors want to know only the design, but later they may question how the authors determined a conclusion, or what a specific subset of patients had for a specific treatment. Having a firm grasp on the methodology allows you to answer many of their questions.

The study design and methodology have been a challenge researchers have had to overcome for treatments such as manipulation. The following is taken from *Manipulative and Body-Based Practices: An Overview*.[3] This report is available from the NCCAM and highlights the difficulty in designing clinical trials.

Clinical trials of CAM manual therapies face the same general challenges as trials of procedure-based interventions such as surgery, psychotherapy, or more conventional physical manipulative techniques (e.g., physical therapy). These include:

- Identifying an appropriate, reproducible intervention, including dose and frequency. This may be more difficult than in standard drug trials, given the variability in practice patterns and training of practitioners.
- Identifying an appropriate control group(s). In this regard, the development of valid sham manipulation techniques has proven difficult.
- Randomizing subjects to treatment groups in an unbiased manner. Randomization may prove more difficult than in a drug trial, because manual therapies are already available to the public; thus, it is more likely that participants will have a preexisting preference for a given therapy.
- Maintaining investigator and subject compliance to the protocol. Group contamination (which occurs when patients in a clinical study seek additional treatments outside the study, usually without telling the investigators; this will affect the accuracy of the study results) may be more problematic than in standard drug trials, because subjects have easy access to manual therapy providers.
- Reducing bias by blinding subjects and investigators to group assignment. Blinding of subjects and investigators may prove difficult or impossible for certain types of manual therapies. However, the person collecting the outcome data should always be blinded.
- Identifying and employing appropriate validated, standardized outcome measures.
- Employing appropriate analyses, including the intent-to-treat paradigm.[3]

Study Participants (the *n*)

Doctors want to know how many participants were in the study. This is commonly referred to as *n*, and a study that has 480 study participants might list it as *n* = 480. The smaller the study group, the more profound the positive findings should be because a higher rate of chance is associated with the outcome. The more patients you have in a study, the more valid the outcome.

The number of study participants can be used to overcome a doctor's objection. For instance, if a doctor were to say to you that he would not prescribe manipulative therapy for a patient with neck pain because it caused a headache in one of his patients in the past, you could professionally overcome this objection by asking the doctor if he would base his other treatments on evidence from a study with only one participant, or a study of *n* = 1. You could also sympathize with the doctor and explain that you had a patient who had vomiting associated with the pain medication prescribed, but that you wouldn't assume that every patient who took the pain medication would have vomiting. Side effects can happen with every therapy. An *n* = 1 is not a fair sample, and it wouldn't mean much in the overall clinical setting. The best way to handle this specific objection is to sympathize and then move on to a study with a large number of patients. In the data, look directly at the number of patients who had a headache associated with cervical manipulation.

Objective Measurements

When it comes to back pain, the objective measurement used to determine efficacy is mainly a subjective pain questionnaire. Doctors are accustomed to using subjective measurement scales to illustrate the efficacy of a treatment. Depending on patients' subjective complaints, the questionnaire can translate that information into a more objective measurement that can be compared at different treatment intervals. The most frequent questionnaires used in the research are listed here and in Appendix G. If you come upon a questionnaire that is not discussed, the Internet is a good reference tool as is Dr. Haneline's book for learning more about it. All of these questionnaires should be available for the doctor to review.

McGill Pain Questionnaire (MPQ)

This questionnaire has stood the test of time and is as popular today as it was more than 30 years ago when it was first introduced. As such, new pain scales are frequently compared to it. As Dr. Haneline indicates, it is the "gold standard" in pain questionnaires.[1] The design was meant to derive a quantitative measure of pain to be used statistically. There is also a short form available that takes less time to administer but offers a similar quantitative analysis. Several Web sites allow you to download this form at no charge. The MPQ has several components that address sensory pain, affective pain, and intensity of pain. Also included is a pain diagram. Grading of the short form is straightforward. For sensory, add together the corresponding scores and divide by the number of questions for each section (mild = 1, moderate = 2, severe = 3, no answer = 0). Sensory is covered in questions 1 through 11. Affective is covered in questions 12 through 15. To gather the overall mean score add all answers together and divide by 15.

Oswestry Disability Index (ODI)

The ODI or Oswestry Low Back Pain Disability Questionnaire has been around for many years and is considered the gold standard for lower back functional outcome. The test has 10 questions and each answer has a point value associated with it. To score the test all points for the answers provided by the patient are added up, divided by the highest amount of points possible (50), and then multiplied by 100. The score is then evaluated as follows:

> 0% to 20%: Minimal Disability
>
> 22% to 40%: Moderate Disability
>
> 41% to 60%: Severe Disability
>
> 61% to 80%: Crippled
>
> 81% to 100%: Bed-bound or malingering

Roland Morris Questionnaire (RMQ)

The important correlation of the RMQ is that, like the ODI, it has been proven to be reliable over time and it has also been shown to be sensitive over time for lower back pain. The only issue with the RMQ is that there is no associated scale for pain and the related disability. Therefore, this is a questionnaire that must be administered at baseline to quantify pain reduction. There are notations in the literature that indicate a score of 13 or higher is related to poor outcome, and clinically important differences in pain are indicated by a change of 4 or 5 points.

Neck Disability Questionnaire (NDI)

The NDI is similar to the ODI. The questions are related to the neck, and the test is scored and assessed in the same manner as the ODI. The percentage grading system is the same as the ODI for disability levels.

SF-36 (RAND 36-Item Health Survey)

This is not specific to a regional area of the body but rather encompasses the general health of a patient. It is used widely in research but has been adapted for clinical use as well. It is popular in overseas studies as a benchmark. There are eight components of the questionnaire:

1. Limits in physical activities as a result of overall health
2. Limits in role of activities as a result of overall health
3. Bodily pain
4. General health
5. Vitality
6. Limits in social activities because of physical or emotional problems
7. Limits in usual role of social activities because of physical or emotional problems.
8. Mental health

Scoring this test is not as easy as the others, and thus it is not as widely utilized in everyday practice.

The Visual Analog Scale and the Numeric Rating Scale

Each of these tests consists of a scale that is easy to administer and easy for the patient to answer. The scales have a no pain to worst pain range, or 0 = No Pain to 10 = Worst Pain. They are both used in clinical practice and in research.

The Bournemouth Questionnaire (BQ)

This questionnaire was developed by the Anglo European Chiropractic College (AECC). This questionnaire has not been utilized in research that is included in this text; however, it appears to have the potential to make an appearance in future research and is included here for reference. The following is taken from the AECC Web site as a description of the test and its use:

> The . . . BQ was developed . . . for use to monitor outcomes in patients with musculoskeletal pain. It is a multidimensional instrument based on the dimensions of the biopsychosocial model of pain and is short enough to be practical for use in the busy clinical setting. It has been validated in back pain (*Journal of Manipulative and Physiological Therapeutics* 1999; 22:503–510) and neck pain (*Journal of Manipulative and Physiological Therapeutics* 2001;25:141–148) patients. . . . The BQ comes in two parts:

the first is the pre-treatment questionnaire, which is for use at the start of treatment and includes demographic and clinical details: the second is the post-treatment questionnaire for use throughout treatment at those time points you feel appropriate to measure outcomes. The BQ is scored by totaling the scores of the seven dimensions and giving as either a total score or converting to a percentage score ((score/70) × 100).[4]

The *p* Value

Two terms to be familiar with are *significant* and *statistically significant*. To be statistically significant a finding of two study groups (either head to head or treatment vs. control group) must have an assigned *p* (probability) value of < .05 percent and that means that the differences between the groups are unlikely to be due to chance. The larger the difference between groups, the less likely it is that it's due to chance. *P* values range from 0 to 1, with 0 meaning that there was no chance, and 1 meaning certainty. A *p* value of .05 is better than a *p* value of .10 because it means 1 out of 20 patients may have had a false positive versus 1 out of 10. As you look at the tables presented in studies, note the asterisk next to some values. Look at the legend to determine what the authors assigned as the *p* value.

Conclusions

There really isn't much to explain here except the obvious. It is desirable to have positive conclusions, but watch out for conclusions that have the appearance of being overly biased or exceptionally in favor of a treatment. Conclusions should be based on facts with no inference drawn from the data. They are simple and straightforward.

Reference Sections

The Reference section listed at the end of a research paper is also something to take into consideration but not something from which you would promote. If you note in the Reference section a high usage of a particular research paper, it is worth your time to investigate whether that is another potential paper to use for promotional purposes. The references lend credibility to a research paper; for instance, a research paper that uses primarily negative references on manipulation could be construed as biased and the paper loses credibility, and vice versa.

The studies included in this text are presented in the following format:

Title and Authors: The title of the study, authors, publication name, and publication date are listed.

Proof Source: The listings under this heading allow you to quickly determine what the paper can best be utilized for. For instance: safety, cost, efficacy on lower back, and so on.

Abstract: This is an exact copy of the abstract as it appears in the original publication and is intended to provide you with an overview of the study.

Promotional Strengths: Key points of the studies are listed. *Key points* are defined as those points in the study that could be illustrated in a promotional setting. This section focuses on setting up the study, including journal name, publication date, number of participants, and study design. In addition, this section lists tables and graphs that would appeal to the medical community and makes highlighting the data quick and easy. The graphs are not reproduced in the body of this text. I suggest that if the highlights of the study appeal to you, you should secure a copy of the article and read the article along with the points made in this book. If you are a member of the ACA or subscribe to *JMPT*, obtaining a copy of the article will not be too expensive. Prior to presenting the article, rehearse so that you can recite all of the pertinent information as well as an overview of the findings without looking at the study itself. This will also enable you to become familiar enough with the study to recall it as a source when you are in a promotional setting. Finally, this section is not a strict outline of what you should and should not promote. You may find other points in the study that you feel are worthy of promoting. If 10 chiropractors reviewed a clinical study for its promotional strengths, there would be 10 variations of how the study should be presented. Some doctors will respond to some of the graphs and key points and others won't. In addition, some doctors won't want you to cover every key point but would rather have a quick illustration of one or two tables and key points.

Potential Questions and Objections: This section will alert you to possible objections by the doctor relative to the study along with a strategy to overcome the objection or another proof source to use to overcome or clarify the objection. Do not confuse this with a strategy to "spin" data in your favor during a promotional opportunity. It is just that if there is another credible proof source or viewpoint that can overcome a paper's weakness, it will be pointed out in this section.

Patient Type: This section provides an example of what type of patient picture to paint for the physician that is supported by the research.

Bottom Line: If you had only a minute to summarize this paper for a doctor, the bottom line section provides a concise summary statement to help you make your point.

The research that is included in this text is research that can be promoted with medical doctors. The reason each study is included varies. The strengths and weaknesses of the study are explained, again from a promotional perspective. Strategies to present these papers and key points are pointed out. You may choose to use other studies, and I encourage you to do so with a precautionary warning to stick with the preceding guidelines on what makes a credible study.

For this book, the cutoff date for references was May 2007 for all chapters except Chapter 9 on safety. Chapter 9 is current through September 2007 simply because of the importance of this chapter. References for this book will be updated on Aligned Methods, or you can perform literature searches for new information.

REFERENCES

1. Haneline MT. *Evidence-Based Chiropractic Practice.* 1st ed. Sudbury, MA: Jones and Bartlett; 2007.

2. Sackett DL, Rosenberg WM, Gray JA, Haynes RB, Richardson WS. Evidence-based medicine: what it is and what it isn't. *Br Med J.* 1996;312(7023):71–72.

3. National Center for Complementary and Alternative Medicine. *Manipulative and Body-Based Practices: An Overview.* Bethesda, MD: National Center for Complementary and Alternative Medicine; October 2004. NCCAM Publication No. D238.

4. Anglo European Chiropractic College. Bournemouth Questionnaire. Available at http://www.aecc.ac.uk/research/bmth_questionnaire/index.asp. Accessed January 9, 2008.

Chapter 7

Chiropractic's Key Selling Points

Having defined how to gather key research with a firm grasp on the promotional selling strategies, we can turn our focus to your first meeting with a physician in which the primary objective is to examine chiropractic's strengths and market value. The first sales encounters with physicians won't necessarily be competitive, but they will be informative. This chapter looks at presenting the facts on chiropractic, which can be summarized through key selling points.

Key selling points are those characteristics that provide value in a service. Adding value is critical. The entire chiropractic industry needs to illustrate its value as an integral provider of back pain treatment if it is to remain a viable component of health care with managed care coverage.

Currently, the majority of articles that address back pain fail to mention chiropractors as valuable treatment providers for lower back pain, a condition for which chiropractic has been proven to be both effective and cost-effective. Hospitals and large medical groups that add holistic care look to massage therapy and acupuncture and often fail to consider chiropractors as an integral member of the healthcare team. The general healthcare community knows that chiropractors treat back pain but clearly don't understand the value chiropractors bring in treating one of the most common medical conditions. More disappointing is that chiropractic excels as a holistic treatment approach with high rates of efficacy for a condition with limited treatment options. An added bonus is that chiropractic is covered by insurance, which decreases patients' out-of-pocket expenses.

Typically, the sequence for patients with back pain is to see if the pain resolves by itself, which may or may not include days of lost work and pharmacologic intervention. Then, the patient may be referred for special tests or physical therapy. If the pain persists, the patient is referred to an orthopedic surgeon, with surgery often the final option. Chiropractic care should fit in the beginning of the sequence of treatment, especially because chiropractors' primary tool, manipulation, has been proven to be effective in reducing pain and disability and can prevent the need for orthopedic referral.

The following key selling points are adapted from the World Federation of Chiropractic and explain how chiropractic services can add value to health care and patients.

Chiropractic's Key Selling Points

- Chiropractors are the spinal healthcare experts in the healthcare system.
- Chiropractic has the ability to improve function in the neuromusculoskeletal system, and overall health, well-being, and quality of life.
- Chiropractic is a specialized approach to examination, diagnosis, and treatment based on best available research and clinical evidence, and with particular emphasis on the relationship between the spine and the nervous system.
- Chiropractic has a tradition of effectiveness and patient satisfaction.
- Chiropractic is a conservative, clinical, safe treatment approach without the use of drugs and surgery, enabling patients to avoid these when possible.
- Chiropractic has proven cost-effectiveness in the managed care, workers' compensation, and Medicare markets.
- Chiropractors are expertly qualified providers of spinal adjustment, manipulation and other manual treatments, exercise instruction, and patient education.
- Chiropractors collaborate with other health professionals.
- Chiropractic is a patient treatment approach focusing on individual responsibility for health, encouraging patient independence.
- Chiropractors are expert, professional, ethical, knowledgeable, and compassionate healthcare providers.[1]

In a sales call, mention a few of the key selling points of chiropractic in a conversational manner. Each key point provides you with a starting place for a conversation, and each can be related to the promotional material found within this text. In presenting chiropractic care to a physician for the first time, you will spend a lot of time ascertaining the physician's current understanding of chiropractic care, in particular his or her understanding of manipulation and its effects on the body. Figure 7–1 is a starting promotional presentation algorithm.

As illustrated, an introduction to chiropractic care and an explanation of the mechanism of action for manipulation are the first steps. From there, discuss which conditions chiropractic is indicated for and that it is covered and

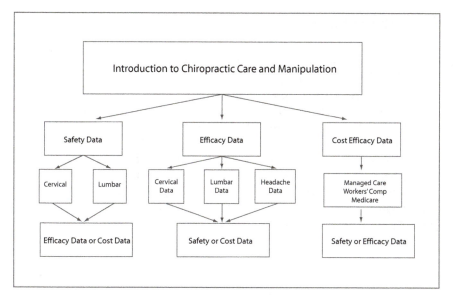

Figure 7–1 *Sales call algorithm.*

available on insurance. Mentioning insurance that mirrors the insurance the doctor sees in his or her own practice will add impact to your presentation. Next, ask the doctor what material he or she is interested in to lead you further into the sales algorithm.

This chapter covers the basic mechanism of action of manipulation that will help you illustrate the science supporting our most valuable treatment tool. This is one of the most important parts of your presentation. Not only are you illustrating research, but you are also educating the physician on a new treatment option. Although this part of the presentation is anatomically in-depth, you do not have to get extremely technical. The medical community must understand how manipulation works if the rest of the research is to make any sense. The following research paper does a nice job of providing a mechanism of action of manipulation.[2]

"Review: Mechanism of Action of Spinal Manipulative Therapy." Jean-Yves Maigne, Philippe Vautravers. *Joint Bone Spine.* 2003;70:336–341.

Proof Source

• Mechanism of Action for Manipulation

Abstract

Spinal manipulative therapy (SMT) acts on the various components of the vertebral motion segment. SMT distracts the facet joints, with faster separation when a cracking sound is heard. Intradiscal pressure may decrease briefly. Forceful stretching of the paraspinal muscles occurs, which induces relaxation via mechanisms that remain to be fully elucidated. Finally, SMT probably has an inherent analgesic effect independent from effects on the spinal lesion. These changes induced by SMT are beneficial in the treatment of spinal pain but short-lived. To explain a long-term therapeutic effect, one must postulate a reflex mechanism, for instance the disruption of a pain–spasm–pain cycle or improvement of a specific manipulation-sensitive lesion, whose existence has not been established to date.

Promotional Strengths

- Published in *Joint Bone Spine*
- Recent publication: 2003
- Authors have hospital affiliation (physical medicine)
- Provides an explanation for the mechanism of action of manipulation:
  - Facet joint separation
    Resulting in a release of energy and creating joint cavitation usually with an associated popping noise
  - Stretching of the paraspinal muscle
    Forces muscle relaxation
  - Decreased intradiscal pressure
    Decreasing pressure in the annulus and endplates, which when under pressure may activate nerve endings and cause pain
- Provides further explanation on how this mechanism provides pain relief:
  Effect on pain from three separate mechanisms
  - A rise in plasma beta endorphin (provides an analgesic effect), which has been documented to occur after SMT
  - Activation of the descending pain inhibitory system by stretching structures that make up the vertebral motor unit
  - Muscle stretching that induces afferent presynaptic inhibition, which decreases cutaneous pain, which is known to occur locally after SMT

Potential Questions and Objections

- No clear pictures or diagrams to help facilitate the conversation. Using an MVA or a spine model would be helpful as a visual aid.

Patient Type

- Any patient without contraindication to manipulation

Bottom Line

"The mechanism of action of manipulation is to anatomically separate the facet joints, stretch the paraspinal muscles, and decrease the intradiscal pressure, all of which aid in pain relief and increased mobility."

Some doctors will be very interested in the science behind manipulation, and several studies will further support the preceding study for a doctor who wants to delve further into the mechanism of action. One such study that focuses on the joints of the spine and the restoration of movement is provided here.[3]

"The Effects of Side-Posture Positioning and Spinal Adjusting on the Lumbar Z Joints: A Randomized Controlled Trial with Sixty-Four Subjects." Gregory Cramer, Douglas Gregerson, J. Todd Knudsen, Bradley Hubbard, Leah Ustas, Joe Cantu. *Spine.* 2002;27(22):2459–2466.

Proof Source

- Effects of Side Posturing on the Lumbar Joints

Abstract

Study Design. A blinded, randomized controlled trial was conducted.

Objective. To test the hypothesis that chiropractic side-posture manipulation (adjusting) of the lumbar spine separates (gaps) the zygapophysial (Z) joints.

Summary of Background Data. Spinal adjusting is thought to gap the Z joints, yet no studies have conclusively validated this hypothesis, and some investigators have reported that the lumbar Z joints do not gap during rotation.

Methods. For this study, 64 healthy student volunteers (32 men and 32 women) ages 22 to 30 years with no history of significant low back pain were randomized into four groups of 8 men and 8 women each. Interventions included lumbar side-posture spinal adjusting (manipulation) and side-posture positioning. Anterior to posterior measurements of the Z joints from MRI scans taken before and after side-posture spinal adjusting and before and after side-posture positioning were compared.

Results. Observers performing the measurements were blinded as to group and first and second scans. Reliability of the measurements was established. Differences were found between the groups (F = 24.15; P < 0.000, analysis of variance). Side-posture positioning showed greater gapping than the control condition (mean difference, 1.18; P < 0.000); side-posture adjusting showed greater gapping than the control condition (mean difference, 1.89; P < 0.000), and side-posture adjusting showed greater gapping than side-posture positioning (mean difference, 0.71; P = 0.047).

Conclusions. Spinal adjusting produced increased separation (gapping) of the Z joints. Side-posture positioning also produced gapping, but less than that seen with lumbar side-posture adjusting. This study helps to increase understanding about the mechanism of action for spinal manipulation.

Promotional Strengths

- Published in *Spine*
- Recent publication: 2002
- Supports the mechanism of action of manipulation and illustrates a distinct physical change confirmed by magnetic resonance imaging (MRI).
- For a doctor who is skeptical of manipulation and how it works, this adds more scientific data to your promotional efforts

Potential Questions and Objections

- Small group of study participants
  - Despite this, the evidence seems fairly clear from MRIs before and after manipulation that gapping of the Z joints does occur.

Patient Type

- Not necessarily a patient type, this paper supports the Maigne paper.

Bottom Line

> "Patients who undergo side-posture manipulation had gapping in their Z joints that was not present prior to manipulation based on pre and post MRIs."

This study serves as an example that if you can't get buy-in from a doctor using Maigne's mechanism of action paper, you can try to ascertain the specific point of the objection and provide the literature that supports the science to which the doctor is objecting.

Deciding What to Promote Next

Once you have explained the mechanism of action of manipulation, it is important in a promotional setting to try to understand what data you might want to present next. Asking the doctor for feedback on the mechanism of action may bring up questions on safety or questions on what conditions manipulation is appropriate for. If, for example, the doctor asks about safety, make sure you qualify exactly what kind of safety data he or she is looking for. Don't assume it is for the cervical region; rather, simply ask if he or she is interested in safety data on the neck, lumbar region, or both. You can then move into a study that examines safety.

If the doctor asks about patient conditions, it is a wonderful opportunity to probe the doctor for conditions commonly seen in his or her practice that can further be used to set up patient types when presenting studies. Keep in mind that the question the doctor asks may not necessarily be covered by a specific study but rather by a group of studies. For instance, the doctor may inquire about the number of visits needed to resolve a particular condition. Ask if the doctor is interested in knowing the answer for patients with acute or chronic lower back pain, headaches, neck pain, or other. Once you have the answer, you can then move to a study or a group of studies that covers these conditions and point out the average number of visits. From there, you can ask probing questions on the data, such as: "Doctor, you were interested in the safety of lumbar manipulation. Does this mean you have a lot of patients with lower back pain?"

An affirmative answer can then lead you to move into the efficacy data for the lumbar regions. The opportunities are endless, and making sure to tie the study to the doctor's interest and patient's, as well as asking probing questions, will yield you a bounty of endless promotional opportunities.

There are two items you will want to point out consistently in each study:

- "No serious adverse events" (even if you are discussing efficacy)
- "Patient satisfaction"

Both of these are fairly consistently noted in most studies. Getting in the habit of summarizing the study and including these points is important.

There are five key components in promoting manipulation:

1. The mechanism of action of manipulation
2. The safety of manipulation
3. The efficacy of manipulation
4. The cost efficacy of chiropractic care
5. The overall patient satisfaction associated with chiropractic care

Although there is research specifically related to patient satisfaction, it is better to be proactive with your time with the physician and mention patient satisfaction as it is related in the research studies that you are utilizing rather than dedicating precious time to just patient satisfaction.

Clearing Up the Misconceptions

Most doctors have concerns surrounding chiropractic care as follows:

- Amount and frequency of care or "failure of chiropractors to treat and release"
  - Focus on the number of visits study participants had to get relief. Set up the type of pain and disability the patients had (mild, moderate, severe, acute, chronic, unable to work, and so on). A patient who is better after an average of four visits is not meaningful unless the doctor can correlate the specifics of the case to a similar patient in his or her own office. "Patients with moderate neck pain and disability who are better after an average of four visits" is more meaningful a statement than "it takes about four visits." This latter statement can cause confusion and misunderstanding if a doctor believes a patient with severe neck pain could see the same results.
- Safety, primarily of the cervical region
- Conditions that chiropractors treat (treat within scope of practice)
- Cost (not wanting to refer a patient to a chiropractor who overtreats or pushes nutritional or other products)
  - Clarify whether the doctor wants to know about costs in your office, which may include insurance coverage, or whether he or she is asking if you are going to promote accessory products that run up patients' out-of-pocket expenses.
  - This may overlap with the amount of care or office visits needed to resolve a condition.

Looking at Research from a Promotional Standpoint

Keep in mind several important considerations as you review the research disclosed in the next few chapters.

- Manipulation is no longer exclusive to chiropractic, but it is a chiropractor's primary treatment tool. As such, promoting manipulation promotes your practice. It doesn't mean that you should not promote your use of therapeutic ultrasound, massage, and so on. Doctors already accept physical therapy as an appropriate treatment for neuromuscular pain, and you should mention that you can provide it as well if this is true for your practice and state licensing laws.

- The research in this text is limited to empirical and consistent research. This means that at the time of publication, it is focused on the lower back, neck, and headaches. It does not imply that I believe manipulation is not appropriate for other conditions.

- The research focuses on the conditions for which doctors will most likely refer and chiropractors are most likely to treat. As such, because chiropractors treat the majority of patients for lower back and neck pain, these are the conditions that should be promoted. It would be a waste of time to promote a condition that makes up 5 percent of your practice, unless the doctor asks about it.

A Good Starting Point

Once you feel the doctor has a comprehensive understanding of manipulation and the more important issues of chiropractic, you can steer the conversation in a more competitive direction. The goal is to prove that the efficacy of manipulation is at least as effective as the competitor's treatments but has the advantage of safety as well as lower cost. The studies you choose to use depend on the competitor you have identified. Beginning with chronic lower back pain—if you haven't already discussed it—is a great starting point for the following reasons:

- Doctors are not as concerned with the safety of lumbar manipulation.
- Acute lower back pain may be naturally self-limiting.
- Chronic lower back pain accounts for the majority of costs, pain, and disability with few options for treatments. Doctors are ready to refer these patients out, mostly to physical therapists and orthopedic doctors.
- The research supporting manipulation in the treatment of lower back pain is consistent and strong.

These are guidelines to the information that you should strive to present to the doctor in your initial sales calls. The purpose of the first sales call is to educate the doctor on manipulation and other services you can provide to patients with neuromuscular pain. You also want to dispel the myths that are commonly associated with chiropractic care. From there, as we will see in the next few chapters, the opportunities are endless.

REFERENCES

1. World Federation of Chiropractic. www.wfc.org/website/WFC/website.nsf/WebPage/ IdentityConsultation?OpenDocument&ppos=2&spos=4&rsn=y

2. Maigne J, Vautravers P. Review: Mechanism of action of spinal manipulative therapy. *Joint Bone Spine*. 2003;70:336–341.

3. Cramer GD, Gregerson D, Knudsen JT, Hubbard BB, Ustas LM, Cantu JA. The effects of side-posture positioning and spinal adjusting on the lumbar Z joints: a randomized controlled trial with sixty-four subjects. *Spine*. 2002;27(22):2459–2466.

The Evidence for Efficacy of Manipulation

T his chapter looks at some of the more recent clinical trials on the efficacy of manipulation in the treatment of headaches as well as issues of
the lumbar and cervical regions. Although there is promising evidence
for the treatment of conditions such as carpal tunnel syndrome, such information is not included because the evidence is simply not consistent at
the time of publication. The intentions of this text are to provide you with
conditions and the associated research that you can promote with absolute
confidence; if one proof source or study doesn't hit home with the physician,
there is an alternate study to turn to. If you were to present a study on a condition such as carpal tunnel syndrome and the doctor objected to your proof
source, you would have limited resources to turn to for another proof source.
This not only destroys your credibility but in this doctor's eyes simply
serves as proof that the chiropractic profession is not yet legitimate or that
the research is still young and not conclusive. In addition, chiropractors
spend 95% of their time on the back, and the time you spend promoting
should be spent promoting the major conditions that chiropractors see in
their offices every day.

This is not to say that if a doctor were to ask you for information on carpal
tunnel that you can't present it. It would be logical for a doctor to understand
the concept of the effect of manipulation on neuromuscular conditions and
then ask how it pertains to carpal tunnel syndrome. In this case, you can
explain to the doctor that the research is just coming along and looks promising. Ask if you can pull the research that is available and even discuss your
treatment approach for carpal tunnel syndrome. This will make more impact
and provide a straightforward approach to sharing this evidence.

For the purposes of this text, the conditions that have multiple proof
sources and empirical evidence are provided as examples in this text. The

efficacy studies included in this chapter are all available on common medical search engines and printed in reputable journals, as highlighted in Chapter 6. The numbers of study participants are acceptable and oftentimes impressive, and the results are consistent. The studies presented here have an overall favorable message with sound methodology. Provided you are a member of the American Chiropractic Association, many of these studies will be free for you to review in their entirety and are also cost effective when ordering clinical reprints with which to provide the doctor.

This chapter is split into four sections. The studies listed in this section are in no particular order.

- Lumbar efficacy studies
- Cervical efficacy studies
- Studies that contain both lumbar and cervical findings
- Headache studies

Section I: Lumbar Efficacy Studies

There are four clinical articles that make up the UK BEAM Trial (United Kingdom Back pain Exercise And Manipulation). They are the following:

- Spinal Manipulation for Low-Back Pain: A Treatment Package Agreed by the UK Chiropractic, Osteopathy and Physiotherapy Professional Associations
- UK Back pain Exercise And Manipulation (UK BEAM) Trial: National Randomized Trial of Physical Treatments for Back Pain in Primary Care: Objectives, Design and Interventions
- United Kingdom Back pain Exercise And Manipulation (UK BEAM) Randomised Trial: Effectiveness of Physical Treatments for Back Pain in Primary Care
- United Kingdom Back pain Exercise And Manipulation (UK BEAM) Randomised Trial: Cost Effectiveness of Physical Treatments for Back Pain in Primary Care. (This study is in Chapter 10, "Cost-Effectiveness of Chiropractic Care.")

The two latter clinicals are the trial results and will be the ones you want to utilize for promotional purposes. The first two clinicals will add to your understanding of the trial design and may be called upon for a doctor who desires an in-depth explanation of the trial. Because the first two clinicals are not intended to be illustrated in a promotional setting, the promotional strengths, promotional weaknesses, patient types, or bottom line presentations are not presented in this text, but rather key points are highlighted to aid in your understanding of the trial results that are then presented.

"Spinal Manipulation for Low-Back Pain: A Treatment Package Agreed by the UK Chiropractic, Osteopathy and Physiotherapy Professional Associations." E. Harvey, A.K. Burton, J.K. Moffett, A. Breen, in collaboration with the UK BEAM trial team. *Manual Therapy.* 2003; 8(1):46–51.

Proof Source

To aid in the understanding of the methodology and clinical outcomes discussed in the main efficacy trial

Abstract

Summary: Trials of manipulative treatment have been compromised by, amongst other things, different definitions of the therapeutic procedures involved. This paper describes a spinal manipulation package agreed by the UK professional bodies that represent chiropractors, osteopaths and physiotherapists. It was devised for use in the UK Back pain Exercise And Manipulation (UK BEAM) trial, a national study of physical treatments in primary care funded by the Medical Research Council and the National Health Service Research and Development Programme. Although systematic reviews have reported some beneficial effects of spinal manipulation for low-back pain, due to the limited methodological quality of primary studies and difficulties in defining manipulation, important questions have remained unanswered. The UK BEAM trial was designed to answer some of those questions. Early in the design of the trial, it was acknowledged that the spinal manipulation treatment regimes provided by practitioners from the three professions shared more similarities than differences. Because the trial design specifically precluded comparison of the effect between the professions, it was necessary to devise a homogenous package representative of, and acceptable to, all three. The resulting package is "pragmatic," in that it represents what happens to most people undergoing manipulation, and "explanatory" in that it excludes discipline specific variations and other ancillary treatments.

Key Points

Spinal manipulation package:

- Patients would remain with the same practitioner who administered the first treatment (chiropractor or doctor of osteopathy).
- First treatment included an assessment, explanation (not discipline specific), and treatment (including one or more of the proposed treatments within the package).
- Subsequent sessions were about 20 minutes focused on the administration of treatment.
- At the discretion of the practitioner, a maximum of 8 sessions could be spread over the intervention period of 12 weeks (or 6 weeks in the case of the patients enrolled for manipulation and exercise).
- The practitioner could choose from both manual and nonmanual elements.
  - Manual elements included soft tissue techniques, mobilization, and manipulation.
  - Nonmanual elements included exercises, advice, advocate continuance of normal activities, and positive support.
  - Practitioners were not allowed to manipulate the neck or hand out printed educational material (to avoid contradiction with the active management approach), modalities, appliances, or X-rays (these were to be referred back to the general practitioner [GP]).

As the title suggests, this is an in-depth discussion of the trial design. Any questions that you have as you read the actual trial outcomes that aren't answered in the main bulk of those studies can most likely be referenced in this paper. It is not defensible to present a study to a physician without being intimately familiar with the study design. You don't have to know it from memory, but you should have an idea of the answer and be able to quickly reference it in the support material such as the one provided here.

Proof Source

To aid in the understanding of the methodology and clinical outcomes discussed in the main efficacy trial

Key Points

- What did GP care consist of? What is considered "best practices"?
  - All participants continued to be managed by their GPs even if they were randomized to manipulation or the exercise package. GPs were allowed to advocate the *Back Book*. (The research on the *Back Book* available substantiates its value in improving back beliefs about back pain and that it had a positive influence on the patients' outcome. Other trials that assessed the outcomes associated with this type of patient information have produced a modest effect and because of the low cost and ease of providing this type of information it continues to enjoy a place in health care.[1] In fact, it was recently included as being recommended for low back pain patients by the American College of Physicians and the American Pain Society in a Joint Clinical Practice Guideline for lower back pain.[2] For chiropractors who already educate their patients about back pain, the booklet is not as popular and neither is it consistent with a chiropractor's viewpoint of treating back pain.) Patients were also encouraged by their GPs to remain active. Pain medications were allowed but restricted to analgesics and nonsteroidal anti-inflammatory drugs (NSAIDs). The GPs were discouraged from referring study participants to other physical therapists or specialists during the initial 3 months. It is not clear how many patients needed to continue medication and dosing.
- What did the manipulation package consist of?
  - This was answered earlier in the description of the previous study.
- What did the exercise package consist of?
  - The detailed program was called "The Back to Fitness" program. It is based on the principles of circuit training and incorporates a cognitive-behavioral approach. This was a group program consisting of up to 10 participants per class lasting approximately 1 hour. The classes took place twice a week over 4 weeks, but the option to schedule them over a 12-week period did exist.

- What did the combination package consist of?
  - The purpose of this treatment group was to identify if a more beneficial treatment effect could be gained. As the authors note: "For example, theoretically the combination of manipulation and exercise could be especially beneficial if the exercise maintained any new range of movement gained through manipulation."[3] This treatment group had manipulation for the first 6 weeks followed by exercise for another 6 weeks. This resulted in shorter treatment times for each of the two treatments when compared to the treatments administered by themselves.
- To rule out spontaneous recovery, patients had to have back pain either "28 consecutive days or for at least 21 of these days and at least 21 of the 28 days before that."
- Serious adverse events were monitored and defined as those that occurred that led to hospitalization or death within one week of treatment within the trial. Health professionals (including GPs) were asked to identify any potential adverse events. Patients had follow-up questions at 3 months post treatment and were also asked about hospital admissions; finally, practice research nurses searched participants' records for hospital discharge summaries. Because neck manipulation was not allowed, this information is more suitable for any concern of adverse events related to lumbar manipulation such as cauda equina or ruptured disc.
- This study included 1,334 participants recruited from 168 practices. Twelve-month follow-up was obtained on 75% of the participants.

"United Kingdom Back pain Exercise And Manipulation (UK BEAM) Randomised Trial: Effectiveness of Physical Treatments for Back Pain in Primary Care." *British Medical Journal.* 2004;329:1381.

Proof Source

- Long-term assessment of efficacy in lower back pain
- Efficacy of manipulation
- Safety of lumbar manipulation
- Head-to-head study that illustrates manipulation is more efficacious than exercises and best care practices and that manipulation was not improved substantially by exercises

Abstract

Objective: To estimate the effect of adding exercise classes, spinal manipulation delivered in NHS or private premises, or manipulation followed by exercise to "best care" in general practice for patients consulting with back pain.

Design: Pragmatic randomised trial with factorial design.

Setting: 181 general practices in Medical Research Council General Practice Research Framework; 63 community settings around 14 centres across the United Kingdom.

Participants: 1,334 patients consulting their general practices about low back pain.

Main outcome measures: Scores on the Roland Morris disability questionnaire at three and 12 months, adjusted for centre and baseline scores.

Results: All groups improved over time. Exercise improved mean disability questionnaire scores at three months by 1.4 (95% confidence interval 0.6 to 2.1) more than "best care." For manipulation the additional improvement was 1.6 (0.8 to 2.3) at three months and 1.0 (0.2 to 1.8) at 12 months. For manipulation followed by exercise, the additional improvement was 1.9 (1.2 to 2.6) at three months and 1.3 (0.5 to 2.1) at 12 months. No significant differences in outcome occurred between manipulation in NHS premises and in private premises. No serious adverse events occurred.

Conclusions: Relative to "best care" in general practice, manipulation followed by exercise achieved a moderate benefit at three months and a small benefit at 12 months; spinal manipulation achieved a small to moderate benefit at three months and a small benefit at 12 months; and exercise achieved a small benefit at three months but not 12 months.

Promotional Strengths

- Published in the *British Medical Journal*.
- Recent publication: 2004.
- Mix of authors including MDs.
- Large study population: $n = 1,334$.
- No serious adverse events (lower back).
- Pragmatic study; doctors should identify with how manipulation could add value to treating lower back pain. In addition, it addresses the issue

of treatment choices at a time when it becomes apparent that the back pain is not resolving on its own.

- Long-term follow-up 75% ($n = 995$) at 12 months.
- Multiple questionnaires to make impact and the ability for doctors to identify with at least one. The Roland Morris Questionnaire was the primary outcome measure.
- Setting in both managed care and private practice (in the end, results were combined because of lack of substantial differences between managed care and private practice).
- Statistical significance is noted throughout the study and in the graphs.
- The study contains graphs that are easy to explain and illustrate.
  - On page 4 of the study, Table 1 provides the patient demographics and baseline scores for each of the different patient groups. Not only is this table useful for painting a patient picture consistent with the study, but also it provides immediate feedback on which outcome measurement the doctor would like to have illustrated for the remainder of the study. If, for instance, the doctor prefers to see the Roland Disability scores, use that study throughout the remainder of your presentation as you highlight the data. The demographics listed in this table suggest that a patient in this study could be described as follows:

    A 40 y.o. female who has back pain that is not resolving on its own. The Roland Disability score for the manipulation-alone + best care group is 8.9 and 9.2 for the exercise + best care treatment group at the time of randomization.

  - On pages 5 and 6, Tables 2, 3, and 4 extrapolate the net benefit from exercise, manipulation, and a combination of exercise and manipulation, respectively. As an example, again look at the Roland-Morris scores and explain the tables in combination as follows:

    "Manipulation alone had statistically significant improvement in the Roland Disability score for the manipulation group both at 3 months at 1.57*** and remained significant at 12 months at 1.01* (illustrated in Table 3, page 5 of this study). The exercise-only group was significant only at 3 months at 1.36** and not at all at 12 months at 0.39 (illustrated in Table 2, page 5 of this study)."

  - Figure 2 on page 6 of this study offers a nice visual aid in which the benefits of manipulation clearly stand out when it comes to decreasing the Roland Disability scores and may be explained as follows: "When examining the four treatment groups, the most robust separation from the baseline Roland Disability scores were the treatment groups that included manipulation."

It is important that one not disregard the fact that in a perfect world, manipulation combined with exercise provided the most benefit, albeit questionable when factoring in the cost, which is examined in Chapter 10. Several additional points in favor of manipulation can be made to the physician utilizing this study such as the following:

"The benefits of adding exercise after manipulation was not significant compared to the manipulation only group. If you have a patient with limited insurance benefits, is the cost of providing exercise warranted? The findings in this study don't suggest that they are worth the extra health care cost, especially for a cash-paying patient or a patient who has a maximum allowable benefit per year." This point can be supported in Chapter 10 with the cost analysis portion of the UK BEAM Trial. "Chiropractors have the capability to administer both manipulation and exercises, and I include exercise as a typical component of any treatment plan."

Potential Questions and Objections

- The providers were not limited to chiropractors.
  - "No, in fact it was open to anyone capable of *providing* manipulation. In our area chiropractors are the profession most noted to provide manipulation as their primary treatment tool, and the training chiropractors receive in their collegiate experience is a primary focus." (The option to illustrate the training and hours chiropractors receive at the collegiate level would be appropriate.)
- The study does not define how many treatments patients had in each treatment group.
  - "No, it did not, but it is known that no more than 8 treatments over 1 month were provided in the manipulation-only group, and some patients may not have needed all 8 visits. Eight treatments over 1 month is a reasonable amount of care. Would you agree?"
- The study does not define the medication dosage or how many patients needed prescription medication during the trial.
  - "No, it did not. Patients who do not improve with treatment will have more reliance on pain medications, and that in itself will provide you with how the patient is progressing with chiropractic manipulation. If the patient is not improving with manipulation after 4 to 6 weeks, we would need to reevaluate the response to treatment. Is that a fair assessment?"

- The main outcome measure for this study seems to be the Roland Disability Scale, which does not have a defined rating scale associated with it.
  - "The average Roland Disability score was 9, which is generally considered to be moderate pain. It is cited by experts in this study that a change of 2.5 points is considered to be clinically important. The fact that scores decreased as did the other scores demonstrates efficacy. Do you agree?" Again, one of the promotional strengths of this study is the diversity in rating scales. If the Roland Disability score doesn't appeal to the doctor, return to Table 1 and see which outcome measure might interest the doctor.
- Who was the author?
  - There is an extensive and diverse list of authorship and collaborators. Having the list printed out is helpful. It is available for downloading from http://www.BMJ.com. It is lengthy but impressive.

Patient Types

- Patients whose back pain is not resolving over time and for whom further intervention such as physical therapy (PT) or exercise may be necessary.
- Patients whose back pain is not resolving and who want holistic treatment.
- Patients who have tried exercises and are still not resolving.
- Patients who can't take medication.
- Patients who risk becoming chronic.

The Bottom Line

"Manipulation provided the greatest response to care for patients with unresolving moderate lower back pain; if cost or time is an issue, manipulation alone provided a greater net benefit than exercise alone."

"A Practice-Based Study of Patients with Acute and Chronic Low Back Pain Attending Primary Care and Chiropractic Physicians: Two-Week to 48-Month Follow-Up." Mitchell Haas, Bruce Goldberg, Mikel Aickin, Bonnie Ganger, and Michael Attwood. *Journal of Manipulative and Physiological Therapeutics.* 2004;27:160–169.

Proof Source

- Chronic lower back pain with radiating pain below the knee.
- Acute and chronic lower back pain.
- Efficacy of chiropractic management over medical management for acute and chronic lower back pain with or without radiation.

Abstract

Objective: This study reports pain and disability outcomes up to 4 years for chiropractic and medical patients with low back pain (LBP) and assesses the influence of doctor type and pain duration on clinical outcomes.

Design: Prospective, longitudinal, nonrandomized, practice-based, observational study.

Setting: Fifty-one chiropractic and 14 general practice community clinics.

Subjects: A total of 2,870 acute and chronic ambulatory patients with LBP of mechanical origin.

Methods: Sixty chiropractic (DC) and 111 general practice (MD) physicians participated. Primary outcomes were pain, using a 100-point visual analogue scale (VAS), and functional disability, using the Revised Oswestry Disability Questionnaire. These were measured at baseline and 8 time points. Regression analysis compared acute and chronic DC and MD patients after correcting for baseline differences in the 4 cohorts.

Results: Most improvement was seen by 3 months and sustained for 1 year; exacerbation was seen thereafter. Acute patients demonstrated greater relief at all time points. A clinically important advantage for chiropractic patients was seen in chronic patients in the short term (> 10 VAS points), and both acute and chronic chiropractic patients experienced somewhat greater relief up to 1 year ($P < .000$). The advantage for DC care was prominent for chronic patients with leg pain below the knee ($P < .001$). More than 50% of chronic patients had over 50 days of pain in the third year.

Conclusion: Study findings were consistent with systematic reviews of the efficacy of spinal manipulation for pain and disability in acute and chronic LBP. Patient choice and interdisciplinary referral should be prime considerations by physicians, policymakers, and third-party payers in identifying health services for patients with LBP.

Key indexing terms: Low Back Pain; Outcomes, Predictors; Chiropractic; Medical Care

Promotional Strengths

- Published in the *Journal of Manipulative and Physiological Therapeutics (JMPT)*.
- Recent publication: 2004.
- Authors include MD/DC/PhD.
- Large study population: $n = 2,870$.
- Study design and clinical setting allow the treatment to illustrate how it affects the patient.
- Long-term clinical trial: 2 weeks to 48 months.
- Familiar outcome questionnaires: VAS and Revised Oswestry
- *Chronic* defined as at least 7 weeks of duration.
- Fair treatment plans
  - MD: Prescription drugs, exercise plan, self-care advice (25% were referred for PT)
  - DC: Spinal manipulative therapy (SMT), PT, exercise plan, self-care advice
- Illustrates the necessity for early intervention in any lower back pain because acute pain patients had greater improvement with decreased intensity and pain.
- Quality figures and tables:
  - Table 1 illustrates patient demographics: "Patients with moderate lower back pain with or without radiating lower back pain in their 40s."
  - Figures 1, 2, and 3 on page 163 of the study all illustrate the main findings in this study, which is: "Patients managed by chiropractors enjoyed a sharper decline both in pain and disability in a short period of time. Of note is the greater degree of separation, for patients with chronic pain who experienced a robust decrease in pain and disability in the first 2 weeks of treatment. Doctor, do you agree that this means your patients would require fewer medications and could also reduce their time on disability?"
  - Figure 5 on page 166 provides an illustration for patients recalling pain days between months 24 and 36. "The amount of pain days recalled is less in the chiropractic groups and noticeably less in the acute chiropractic group, which suggests that seeking care earlier in the onset of back pain provides a more enduring decrease in pain and disability long after the initial bout of pain."
  - Table 3 on page 165 provides the opportunity to separate out a discussion on the benefits of chiropractic management for patients with

leg pain that extends below the knee versus lower back pain without radiation. In the text below Table 3, the authors have provided a concise summary to illustrate the table to a doctor:

"As the primary finding, the data suggest a potentially clinically important advantage for DC care in chronic patients with pain radiating below the knee. Adjusted mean differences range from 18.3 to 21.7 in the first year for pain ($P < 0.001$) and 9.0 to 13.9 over 3 years for disability ($P < 0.01$)."[4]

Potential Questions and Objections

- Patients seem to lose any benefit of treatment after 1 year.
  - "Treating lower back pain is difficult for any healthcare professional, and this study illustrates, as the authors point out, that lower back pain persists far longer than previously thought. Faster and more robust resolution in pain and disability is critical for a patient with chronic lower back pain, especially for those with radiating leg pain past the knee. The patients in the chiropractic groups had the fastest and most robust decrease in pain and disability. The fact that they achieved this without pharmacologic intervention or lengthy physical therapy treatments makes chiropractic a very logical first choice. The impact on decreasing disability also makes for a strong clinical rationale to utilize chiropractic manipulation as a first line therapeutic choice. Do you agree?"
- Acute patients don't appear to gain much more benefit from chiropractic treatment; from a cost perspective, medical care might be more cost-effective.
  - "As the authors note, both acute and chronic patients with lower back pain tend to have reoccurrences. When looking at acute pain patients, the patients who had chiropractic care had fewer days of pain 3 years after the acute episode (illustrated in Figure 5, page 166). From both a direct and indirect cost perspective, limiting pain and disability will ultimately result in the most cost-effective care. In this case chiropractic management had more favorable results in the long term for acute patients."

Patient Types

- Patients with chronic low back pain with or without radiating pain below the knee.
- Patients with acute lower back pain with or without radiating pain below the knee.

Bottom Line

"The advantage in this large, long-term study was for chiropractic management over medical management for chronic lower back pain patients especially those with pain radiating below the knee. The majority of relief was seen at 3 months, and acute patients enjoyed the greatest improvement in reducing moderate lower back pain."

"Patient Characteristics, Practice Activities, and One-Month Outcomes for Chronic, Recurrent Low-Back Pain Treated by Chiropractors and Family Medicine Physicians: A Practice-Based Feasibility Study." Joanne Nyiendo, Mitchell Haas, and Peter Goodwin. *Journal of Manipulative and Physiological Therapeutics.* 2000;23:239–245.

Proof Source

- Chiropractic management of chronic recurrent lower back pain performed better with higher patient satisfaction than with medical management
- Manipulation performed better than NSAIDs
- Patients injured at work
- Patient satisfaction
- Clinical outcomes associated with poor emotional status
- Low number of office visits needed for chiropractic manipulation to prove effective in lower back pain

Abstract

Background: Chronic low-back pain is a significant public health problem for which few therapies are supported by predictable outcomes. In this report, practice activities and 1-month outcomes data are presented for 93 chiropractic patients and 45 medical patients with chronic, recurrent low-back pain.

Design: A prospective, observational, community-based feasibility study involving chiropractors and family medicine physicians.

Setting: Forty private chiropractic clinics, the outpatient clinic of the Department of Family Medicine at Oregon Health Sciences University, and 5 other Portland-area family medicine clinics.

Outcomes Measures: The main outcome measures were pain severity, functional disability, sensory and affective pain quality at 1 month, and patient satisfaction assessed at 7 to 10 days and at 1 month.

Results: Although differences were noted in age, sex, education, and employment, the patients were closely matched at baseline with respect to frequency, severity, and type of low-back pain and the psychosocial dimensions of general health. The treatment of choice for chiropractors was spinal manipulation and physical therapy modalities; for medical physicians anti-inflammatory agents were most frequently used. Chiropractic patients averaged 4 visits, and medical patients averaged 1 visit. On average, chiropractic patients showed improvement across all outcomes: 31% change in pain severity, 29% in functional disability, 36% in sensory pain quality, and 57% in affective pain quality. Medical patients showed minimal improvement in pain severity (6%) and functional disability (1%) and showed deterioration in the sensory (29%) and affective (26%) dimensions of pain quality. Satisfaction scores were higher for chiropractic patients. Outcomes for medical patients were heavily dependent on psychosocial status at baseline.

Conclusion: Patients with chronic low-back pain treated by chiropractors show greater improvement and satisfaction at 1 month than patients treated by family physicians. Nonclinical factors may play an important role in patient progress. Findings from the Health Resources and Services Administration–funded project will include a report on the influence of practice activities, including more frequent visits by chiropractic patients, on the clinical course of low-back pain and patient outcomes.

Promotional Strengths

- Published in *JMPT.*
- Authors are MD/DC/PhD.
- Familiar grading scales: VAS and Oswestry Disability.
- Examines recurrent low-back pain (6 weeks of no pain between episodes).
- Workers' compensation patients: 15% of the patient injuries were job related.
- Low number of office visits (average of four office visits for DC care and one office visit for MD care).
- Table 1 on page 241 illustrates patients in their 40s with recurrent lower back pain.
- Table 2 on page 242 of the study provides a strong visual aid comparing the differences in outcome scores between medical and chiropractic management. In all scores, "Chiropractic care resulted in improvements

of patient pain and disability. However, patients in the medical group, the majority of whom utilized NSAIDs, had limited improvement in pain and disability and actually experienced regression in sensory and affective pain quality scores." (In your copy, highlight the relative percentage values for added visual impact. You should also point out that a negative score reflects improvement.)

- Table 3 on page 242 illustrates: "Patient satisfaction was higher in every category for chiropractors in that patients felt that the chiropractor understood their pain and health concerns, had confidence in the care they received, and were comfortable with the care that was provided."

- Table 4 on page 243 reexamines satisfaction and improvement: "Patient satisfaction and improvement at 1 month continued to be consistently in favor of chiropractic care. In particular the majority of chiropractic patients reported that their pain ranged from much better to about the same compared with the majority of medically managed patients treated with NSAIDs who ranged from a little better to much worse."

Potential Questions and Objections

- Low number of study participants: $n = 138$
  - "True, this is not a large study population; however, it is one of the few to correlate outcomes with the patients' emotional status. I am sure you have patients that are angry and frustrated to be living with chronic pain. The patients in this study who underwent chiropractic care expressed greater patient satisfaction for chiropractic management. This is likely because manipulation proved to be effective for a chronic condition and the impact this makes on a patient's life is significant."

    Note: Tread carefully. It is okay to repeat the study findings, but keep in mind some doctors might take this personally, especially if they feel they work hard on their bedside manner and patient outcomes. To overcome this situation it is important to stress the point that chronic patients who finally get better do so because of the effect manipulation had on their pain, not because you are a more compassionate care provider. Patients would be equally satisfied with their medical doctor for referring them to a chiropractor for this type of care *if* it finally resolves or improves their pain and disability. If they didn't get better, they would probably be dissatisfied with both the medical and chiropractic care!

- Not a study designed to look at efficacy of treatment.
  - "This is not a randomized clinical trial, but it certainly provides an explanation of the effect of patient satisfaction and the improvement

noted in pain and disability irregardless of the psychological elements of back pain."

Patient Types

- Patients with chronic and recurrent low-back pain
- Patients who are frustrated with the outcome of their condition
- Patients who have tried NSAIDs and failed
- Patients who should not take NSAIDs as a first-line treatment

Bottom Line

> *"Patients with chronic recurrent lower back pain do better with chiropractic manipulation than NSAIDs and as such were more satisfied patients."*

"A Randomized Clinical Trial Comparing Chiropractic Adjustments to Muscle Relaxants for Subacute Low Back Pain." Kathryn T. Hoiriis, Bruce Pfleger, Frederic C. McDuffie, et al. *Journal of Manipulative and Physiological Therapy.* 2004;27:388–398.

Proof Source

- Efficacy of manipulation over muscle relaxants for subacute lower back pain
- Efficacy of manipulation in pain and disability for subacute lower back pain

Abstract

Background: The adult lifetime incidence for low back pain is 75% to 85% in the United States. Investigating appropriate care has proven difficult since, in general, acute pain subsides spontaneously and chronic pain is resistant to intervention. Subacute back pain has been rarely studied.

Objective: To compare the relative efficacy of chiropractic adjustments with muscle relaxants and placebo/sham for subacute low back pain.

Design: A randomized, double-blind clinical trial.

Methods: Subjects ($N = 192$) experiencing low back pain of 2 to 6 weeks' duration were randomly allocated to three groups with interventions applied over 2 weeks. Interventions were either chiropractic adjustments with placebo medicine, muscle relaxants with sham adjustments, or placebo medicine with sham adjustments. Visual Analog Scale for Pain, Oswestry Disability Questionnaire, and Modified Zung Depression Scale were assessed at baseline, 2 weeks, and 4 weeks. Schober's flexibility test, acetaminophen usage, and Global Impression of Severity Scale (GIS), a physician's clinical impression used as a secondary outcome, were assessed at baseline and 2 weeks.

Results: Baseline values, except GIS, were similar for all groups. When all subjects completing the protocol were combined ($N = 146$), the data revealed pain, disability, depression, and GIS decreased significantly ($P < 0.0001$); lumbar flexibility did not change. Statistical differences across groups were seen for pain, a primary outcome (chiropractic group improved more than control group), and GIS (chiropractic group improved more than other groups). No significant differences were seen for disability, depression, flexibility, or acetaminophen usage across groups.

Conclusion: Chiropractic was more beneficial than placebo in reducing pain and more beneficial than either placebo or muscle relaxants in reducing GIS.

Promotional Strengths

- Published in *JMPT.*
- Recent publication: 2004.
- Authors were DC/MD/PhD.
- Large study population: $n = 192$ (152 received care and 146 returned for final data collection).
- Double blind randomized clinical trial (manipulation with placebo medication or medication with sham manipulation, or placebo medication with sham adjustments).
- Head-to-head data in which manipulation was more effective than muscle relaxants.
- Subjects and assessors were blinded to interventions; chiropractors were blinded to medical/sham assignment. Statistical analysis was provided by an independent consultant.
- Familiar grading scales: VAS, Oswestry, GIS.

- For subacute pain for which a doctor may opt to utilize muscle relaxants, chiropractic is a better choice.
- Appropriate care of eight visits over 2 weeks.
- Graphs provide visual illustration of statistical significance:
  - Table 2 on page 391 illustrates baseline patients were in their 40s, with 3 weeks of sudden, moderate lower back pain.
  - Figures 1 and 2 on page 394 of the study illustrate statistical significance for the VAS and Oswestry outcomes over the control and medication groups. "Patients who received manipulation showed significant improvement in pain and disability compared to patients who received muscle relaxants."
  - Figure 5 on page 395 illustrates statistical significance in GIS outcome over the medication and control groups. "Not only did the chiropractic group have the highest severity ratings, after 2 weeks they also had statistically significant improvement over the control and medical groups."
  - Table 6 on page 393 illustrates the outcome measures for pain and disability: "You will want to highlight data on this graph to add visual impact."

    "This table provides the exact outcome measures for the three treatment groups over the course of the study. For instance, a consistent decline in pain and disability is noted with all groups for the outcomes, but the changes were more dramatic for the chiropractic treatment group especially when looking at the Visual Analog Scale outcomes. In this outcome chiropractic patients had the highest initial scores among the three groups with a mean score of 4.52, and at the end of the study the chiropractic group had the lowest Visual Analog Scores as well at 1.71."

Potential Questions and Objections

- Short-term study
  - "The pain is subacute, the treatment was effective, the patients were released from care."
- There was no long-term follow-up for efficacy.
  - Clarify this question. *"Do you find that many of your patients who respond initially to care develop exacerbations?"* If the doctor says no, then move on. If he or she says yes, then clarify whether he or she is talking about a chronic or recurrent patient and move on to a study that looks at long-term follow-up of chronic or recurrent

patients. Before introducing a new study, summarize this study with a bottom line statement such as this:

"This study examines the efficacy of manipulation over muscle relaxants for subacute pain. Manipulation is also effective in treating chronic lower back or recurrent lower back pain. One study which examines chronic back pain is "A Practice-Based Study of Patients with Acute and Chronic Low Back Pain Attending Primary Care and Chiropractic Physicians: Two-week to 48-month follow up, . . ."

- Some of these patients had pain for only 2 weeks; they could have just had natural recovery.

  - *"I think that is a fair assessment. That might explain why the placebo or control group recovered as well; however, it doesn't explain why the medication and manipulation groups had a more robust recovery over the control. Would you agree that the sooner patients recover the less risk there is for a patient to become chronic?"*

  Note: All of the preceding weaknesses can be overcome by moving to the study discussed earlier titled "A Practice-Based Study of Patients with Acute and Chronic Low Back Pain Attending Primary Care and Chiropractic Physicians: Two-Week to 48-Month Follow-Up." This study takes a look at the long-term data. Most patients do have recurrences, and the data were favorable for treating pain in the acute to subacute phases to reduce long-term recurrences.

Patient Type

- A patient with a first episode of lumbar pain of sudden onset and characterized as constant and moderate pain with muscle spasm or tightness
- A patient who has limited range of motion, lumbar stiffness, and pain, and who is not recovering on his own and for whom the doctor may be considering muscle relaxants

Bottom Line

"Chiropractic manipulation is not only more effective than muscle relaxants for treating sudden, moderate subacute pain; it is also a less invasive treatment option."

Notes on the medication used: Three relaxants were available: cyclobenzaprine HCl, 5 mg; carisoprodol, 350 mg; methocarbamol, 750 mg. Initial dosing varied; it could be doubled or halved as needed. The brand names for these medications are Flexeril, Soma, and Robaxin. The dosing regimen, although not specifically listed per drug, appeared within the normal usage parameters. A common objection a doctor may have when a drug was not as effective compared to another treatment is that the dose administered was too low to achieve a therapeutic benefit. The fact that manipulation is less invasive with better efficacy makes it a better first line treatment.

"Efficacy of Preventive Spinal Manipulation for Chronic Low-Back Pain and Related Disabilities: A Preliminary Study." Martin Descarreaux, Jean-Sébastien Blouin, Marc Drolet, Stanislas Papadimitriou, and Normand Teasdale. *Journal of Manipulative and Physiological Therapeutics*. 2004;27:509–514.

Proof Source

- A specific patient needing more care than usual

  (Note: The majority of our patients do not need preventative care. The exceptions are patients with permanent disabilities, severe injuries, or other chronic conditions. The overall message doctors should hear is that you "treat and release" almost all of your patients. If you have a shared patient who experiences frequent flare-ups, this study provides a limited reference to utilize to support the extra care, through evidence-based research.)

Abstract

Objective: To document the potential role of maintenance chiropractic spinal manipulation to reduce overall pain and disability levels associated with chronic low-back conditions after an initial phase of intensive chiropractic treatments.

Methods: Thirty patients with chronic nonspecific low-back pain were separated into two groups. The first group received 12 treatments in an intensive 1-month period but received no treatment in a subsequent 9-month period. For this group, a 4-week period preceding the initial phase of treatment was used as a control period to examine the sole effect of time on pain and disability levels. The second group received 12 treatments in an intensive 1-month period and also received maintenance spinal manipulation every 3 weeks for a 9-month follow-up period. Pain and disability levels were evaluated with a visual analog scale and a modified Oswestry questionnaire, respectively.

Results: The 1-month control period did not modify the pain and disability levels. For both groups, the pain and disability levels decreased after the intensive phase of treatments. Both groups maintained their pain scores at levels similar to the postintensive treatments throughout the follow-up period. For the disability scores, however, only the group that was given spinal manipulations during the follow-up period maintained their post-intensive treatment scores. The disability scores of the other group went back to their pretreatment levels.

Conclusions: Intensive spinal manipulation is effective for the treatment of chronic low back pain. This experiment suggests that maintenance spinal manipulations after intensive manipulative care may be beneficial to patients to maintain subjective postintensive treatment disability levels. Future studies, however, are needed to confirm the finding in a larger group of patients with chronic low-back pain.

Promotional Strengths

- Published in *JMPT*.
- Recent publication: 2004.
- Offers the opportunity for discussion for a single chronic lower back pain patient who may benefit from preventative care or a case the doctor referred to you who has the need for more care than is typical. It is not meant to advocate lifetime care, maintenance care, or any situation other than to open the discussion for a complicated case. Table 1 on page 511 illustrates all patients had back pain for at least 5 years.

Potential Questions and Objections

- Small sample size: $n = 30$, 15 received preventative care.
  - In this case, it may not be a major issue simply because the percentage of patients who truly need maintenance care is also small. What this is useful for is to document the rare case that isn't responding as robustly as we might like. The concern would be that the doctor might not refer this type of patient because he or she believes care is not working, when in fact the patient may be benefiting from care. What is important is that it wouldn't be wise to stop care and risk losing the benefits that have been gained, but rather to understand that additional care may be necessary such as an increased yet reasonable number of treatments and

possibly add-on exercises, physical therapy, or medication. Removing a treatment that is having some effect could risk an exacerbation.

- Conflicts with other studies on chronic lower back pain in which no preventative treatment was administered and long-term efficacy was documented.
  - This study is reserved for the unusual and more complicated patient. Some patients need more care than others. The UK BEAM trial also documented the need for some patients to seek some form of treatment in the long-term follow-up. This would be an additional proof source when discussing a patient who hasn't failed treatment but who is requiring more treatment than expected.

Patient Types

- A specific patient who is experiencing exacerbations of his symptoms after an initial treatment period of chronic lower back pain

Bottom Line

"A patient who is responding to care at a slower rate may not be failing care and may benefit from extra treatments or additional therapies." or

"Patients in chronic pain may need additional care for flare-ups to return them to their stable pain levels."

It is not appropriate to promote to doctors a regimen that advocates lifetime preventative care, unless there is a reason to substantiate the claim such as a worsening of a chronic condition in which manipulation can relieve the pain back to a certain stable level. There is limited information at this time as to the effectiveness of maintenance care; however, studies are currently being conducted for preventative care for the geriatric population, the findings of which have not yet been released.

Section II: Cervical Studies

"Manual Therapy, Physical Therapy, or Continued Care by a General Practitioner for Patients with Neck Pain; a Randomized, Controlled Trial." Jan Lucas Hoving, Bart W. Koes, Henrica C.W. de Vet, et al. *Annals of Internal Medicine.* 2002;136:713–722.

Proof Source

- Neck pain of recent onset
- Headaches with associated neck pain
- Head-to-head randomized, controlled trial (RCT) of manual therapy, physical therapy and GP care for neck pain
- Side effects of mobilization and PT treatments are similar to those associated with manipulation.

Abstract

Background: Neck pain is a common problem, but the effectiveness of frequently applied conservative therapies has never been directly compared.

Objective: To determine the effectiveness of manual therapy, physical therapy, and continued care by a general practitioner.

Design: Randomized, controlled trial.

Setting: Outpatient care setting in the Netherlands.

Patients: 183 patients, 18 to 70 years of age, who had had nonspecific neck pain for at least 2 weeks.

Intervention: 6 weeks of manual therapy (specific mobilization techniques) once per week, physical therapy (exercise therapy) twice per week, or continued care by a general practitioner (analgesics, counseling, and education).

Measurements: Treatment was considered successful if the patient reported being "completely recovered" or "much improved" on an ordinal six-point scale. Physical dysfunction, pain intensity, and disability were also measured.

Results: At 7 weeks, the success rates were 68.3% for manual therapy, 50.8% for physical therapy, and 35.9% for continued care. Statistically significant differences in pain intensity with manual therapy compared with continued care or physical therapy ranged from 0.9 to 1.5 on a scale of 0 to 10. Disability scores also favored manual therapy, but the differences among groups were small. Manual therapy scored consistently better than the other two interventions on most outcome measures. Physical therapy scored better than continued care on some outcome measures, but the differences were not statistically significant.

Conclusions: In daily practice, manual therapy is a favorable treatment option for patients with neck pain compared with physical therapy or continued care by a general practitioner.

Promotional Strengths

- Published in *Annals of Internal Medicine.*
- Recent publication: 2002.
- Authors were MDs/PTs/ PhDs.
- Study participants: $n = 183$.
- No serious adverse events (cervical).
- Randomized controlled study and head-to-head data of manual therapy, PT, and GP management. (Research assistants were blinded to the type of intervention; 7% of patients accidentally revealed the treatment.)
  - Manual therapy included hands-on muscular mobilization, specific articular mobilization techniques (low-velocity passive movements within the joint range) to improve joint mobility and function. Patients were scheduled for 45 minutes, 1 time a week for 6 weeks.
  - PT included primarily active exercises as well as manual traction, massage, heat, and interferential treatment. Patients were scheduled for 30 minutes, twice a week for a maximum of 12 visits.
  - Continued care by a GP included advice, informational booklet on exercises and ergonomics, and medications including NSAIDs. Patients were seen once with an optional 10-minute visit every 2 weeks. Referrals were discouraged.
- Familiar outcome measure (Numerical Rating Scale, Neck Disability Index [NDI]).
- Figure 1 on page 716 of the study offers a nice flowchart to walk the doctor through the study design.
  - "183 patients were randomly assigned to three separate treatments of manual therapy, physical therapy, and a continued care group. All groups had additional treatments with manual therapy having 5 referred to a general practitioner consultation and 1 for additional exercise; physical therapy had 7 referred to a general practitioner consultation and 1 had an additional treatment of ultrasound; the continued care group referred 6 patients for manual therapy, 1 for physical therapy, 2 for manipulation, and 3 for exercises."
- Table 1 on page 717 of the study illustrates the following patient demographics:
  - Patients with nontraumatic acute or subacute neck pain, history of neck pain, who were primarily females in their early to mid-40s. Half had pain that was bothersome enough to take analgesic medication.
  - Patients had minimal disability. This allows you the opportunity to insert yourself into a treatment option early on before the patient is

subacute or chronic and illustrates that manipulation is effective early on.

- ■ Fifty percent of the patients had headaches in the manual therapy group, and more than 50% had headaches in the PT and continued care groups.
- Table 2 on page 718 displays the adverse reactions, which illustrated that patients had increased neck pain and headaches more notably in the manual therapy and PT groups. This is important because manual therapy is not "manipulation" therapy. This means that adverse events that are associated with manipulation are also associated with any manual or physical treatment to the cervical region, making this a good proof source that manipulation, manual therapy, and PT can all cause a temporary increase in pain and that these adverse events are not limited only to manipulation. The adverse events were described as minor and benign by the authors.
- Figure 2 on page 719 addresses the outcomes (NDI, average pain score, severity of physical dysfunction, and perceived recovery) of treatment for each of the three patient treatment groups. Notably: "Despite the higher incidence of minor adverse events in the physical therapy and manual therapy groups, these two groups had better patient outcomes at the end of treatment especially when it came to comparing manual therapy to continued care."
- Table 3 on page 720 provides more information to support the outcomes of manual therapy compared to continued care. Of note: "The perceived recovery percentage was 68.3% for manual therapy and only 35.9% for continued care, almost two times better."
- PT treatment in this group closely mimics PT in the United States.

Potential Questions and Objections

- Spinal manipulation (high-velocity, low-amplitude thrusts) were not included in this study.
  - ■ If your practice philosophy is no PT, no massage, no soft tissue work or in other words "high-velocity adjustment only," this study will not support the service you are promoting to the physician.
  - ■ If your practice philosophy supports these treatments and your office has the necessary equipment, this study supports the services that you can offer for the physician's patients. In particular, a doctor who resists cervical manipulation may feel more comfortable referring patients to you for this type of patient protocol. It would be important

to continue to educate the physician on cervical manipulation and relative safety for those few patients who may need manipulation if mobilization fails to impact their pain.

- Manual therapy was performed by physical therapists; chiropractors did not participate in this study.
    - Again, if you can provide the services described in this study, this should not be a factor. At least if you provide the care, the patient who does not respond to mobilization does not need another referral for manipulation—you can provide the manipulation.
- The differences between treatments were not large.
    - "The differences between the manual therapy and continued care groups had a significant finding when looking at the perceived recovery. The differences were not as great when looking at disability, but these were acute patients and the baseline disability scores were rated as mild disability to begin with. The dramatic impact is for the effect on pain and perceived recovery for a new episode of pain, to avoid fear avoidance behavior and chronicity."

Patient Types

- Patients with minimal disability who may be a candidate for PT because of nonresolving neck pain.
- Patients who have minimal disability and are not responding to PT care.
- Patients with headaches of a cervical origin (or any other symptom you choose to highlight that is listed in Table 1 such as neck stiffness). The point is to paint a picture of a patient complaint that the doctor may have heard of recently or is likely to hear of in the future that will have him reflect on your treatment as a potential option for that patient.
- Patients who are on multiple medications or have a risk associated with taking NSAIDs.

Bottom Line

"Patients with neck stiffness and pain of recent onset can benefit from mobilization services, which improved range of motion, muscle soreness, and stiffness."

Note: There is an accompanying cost-effectiveness or economic analysis that was done with this trial. The study is listed in Chapter 10.

It is expected that doctors' objections to cervical spine manipulation will be related to safety. As such, safety data may be the first item they want to discuss before they can consider the efficacy data. It would be advisable to ask the doctors which data they would be more interested in reviewing first when it comes to the cervical spine. The safety data is incorporated in Chapter 9.

"A Randomized Trial of Chiropractic Manipulation and Mobilization for Patients with Neck Pain: Clinical Outcomes from the UCLA Neck-Pain Study." Eric L. Hurwitz, Hal Morgenstern, Philip Harber, Gerald F. Kominski, Fei Yu, and Alan H. Adams. *Am Journal of Public Health.* 2002;92:1634–1641.

Proof Source

- Efficacy of manipulation and mobilization for mild to moderate subacute and chronic neck pain
- Headaches with associated neck pain

Abstract

Objectives: This study compared the relative effectiveness of cervical spine manipulation and mobilization for neck pain.

Methods: Neck-pain patients were randomized to the following conditions: manipulation with or without heat, manipulation with or without electrical muscle stimulation, mobilization with or without heat, and mobilization with or without electrical muscle stimulation.

Results: Of 960 eligible patients, 336 enrolled in the study. Mean reductions in pain and disability were similar in the manipulation and mobilization groups through 6 months.

Conclusions: Cervical spine manipulation and mobilization yield comparable clinical outcomes.

Promotional Strength

- Published in *American Journal of Public Health.*
- Recent publication: 2002.
- Authors were DC/MD/PhD.

- Large study population: $n = 336$.
- Page 1638 of the study indicates that there were no known adverse related events and includes a notation that patients in the manipulation arm had more transient and minor discomfort.
- RCT.
- Familiar outcome scales (Numerical Rating Scale, NDI, SF-36).
- Treatments consisted of the following:
  - Chiropractors performing manipulation: high-velocity, low-amplitude thrust. Heat was added prior to manipulation in one group but not in the other.
  - Chiropractors performing mobilization: low-velocity, variable-amplitude movement within passive range of motion.
  - Heat/electrical muscle stimulation (EMS)/Heat and EMS applications: In addition to manipulation or mobilization, patients randomized to receive heat, EMS, or a combination received the therapy prior to mobilization or manipulation. EMS and heat were administered simultaneously.
- Table 1 on page 1636 of the study allows you to set up a patient type:
  - "Patients in this study tended to be female between the ages of 40 to 60 years, with good to excellent health; half of these patients had pain present more than a year. Patients had an NDI consistent with mild to moderate pain, and two-thirds of the patients complained of headaches. Arm pain was present in almost half of the patients, and 40% complained of arm tingling within the past week."
- Figure 1 on page 1638 of the study provides a nice visual aid illustrating: "Both manipulation and mobilization resulted in a dramatic decrease in pain and disability levels primarily in the first 2 to 6 weeks of care."
- Page 1640 of they study includes a section on the complication rates: "Complications are higher for medication and surgery than they are for manipulation and mobilization." If treatments yield a similar outcome, it comes down to which treatment is safer and therefore a more appropriate treatment to begin with.

Potential Questions and Objections

- "You're a chiropractor. This study does not illustrate manipulation."
  - As was seen in the prior study by Hoving et al., mobilization was effective at reducing neck pain and disability.[5] There was no indication that manipulation was statistically significantly better than mobilization. There is every reason for a doctor to want mobilization over

manipulation simply because it is slightly safer. This would also be in accordance with evidence-based health care. If treatments yield the same or similar result, it comes down to which one is safer. While chiropractors frequently utilize manipulation, it is not our only therapeutic treatment tool.

Patient Types

- Patients with moderate chronic or subacute neck pain who may also have headaches, arm pain, or arm numbness

Bottom Line

"Manipulation and mobilization are both effective tools the chiropractor can use to effectively treat moderate neck pain and associated headaches."

Section III: Studies That Contain Both Lumbar and Cervical Findings

"Chiropractic Care of Musculoskeletal Disorders in a Unique Population Within Canadian Community Health Centers." Michael J. Garner, Peter Aker, Jeff Balon, et al. *Journal of Manipulative and Physiological Therapeutics.* 2007;30:165–170.

Proof Source

- Efficacy of chiropractic care in difficult-to-treat patients because of coexisting health conditions and demographic barriers
- Safety in a difficult-to-treat population and those who have coexisting health conditions

Abstract

Objective: This study was part of a larger demonstration project integrating chiropractic care into publicly funded Canadian community health centers. This pre/post study investigated the effectiveness of chiropractic care in reducing pain and disability as well as improving general health status in a unique population of urban, low-income, and multiethnic patients with musculoskeletal (MSK) complaints.

Methods: All patients who presented to one of two community health center–based chiropractic clinics with MSK complaints between August 2004 and December 2005 were recruited to participate in this study. Outcomes were assessed by a general health measure (Short Form-12), a pain scale (VAS), and site-specific disability indexes (Roland-Morris Questionnaire and Neck Disability Index), which were administered before and after a 12-week treatment period.

Results: Three hundred twenty-four patients with MSK conditions were recruited into the study, and 259 (80.0%) of them were followed to the study's conclusion. Clinically important and statistically significant positive changes were observed for all outcomes (Short Form-12: physical composite score mean change = 4.9, 95% confidence interval [CI] = 3.8–6.0; VAS: current pain mean change = 2.3, 95% CI = 1.9–2.6; Neck Disability Index: mean change = 6.8, 95% CI = 5.4–8.1; Roland-Morris Questionnaire: mean change = 4.3, 95% CI = 3.6–5.1). No adverse events were reported.

Conclusions: Patients of low socioeconomic status face barriers to accessing chiropractic services. This study suggests that chiropractic care reduces pain and disability as well as improves general health status in patients with MSK conditions. Further studies using a more robust methodology are needed to investigate the efficacy and cost-effectiveness of introducing chiropractic care into publicly funded health care facilities.

Promotional Strengths

- Published in *JMPT.*
- Recent publication: 2007.
- Mixture of authors: MD/DC/PhD/MSc, and Pran Manga, a prominent Canadian health economist.
- Large study population: $n = 259$.
- No adverse events occurred (cervical and lumbar).
- Familiar outcome measures: VAS, NDI, Roland-Morris, SF-12.
- Funded by the Ontario Ministry of Health and Long-Term Care.
- Table 1 on page 166 of the study identifies patient characteristics:
    - "Patients were primarily females between the ages of 30 and 60 years (other studies have the majority of patients aged 40 to 60; it is interesting to see a higher number of patients in their 30s), with chronic

(> 3 months' duration) lower back pain. Approximately 60% of patients had an annual household income of less than $20,000 in 2004 (Canadian dollars; just under the Canadian poverty line for 2004)."

- Tables 2, 3, and 4 on page 167 of the study illustrate: "Statistical significance and clinical importance in pain, disability, and overall health improvement were observed in the manipulation groups."
- Patient satisfaction is available on page 168 of the study.
  - "Patients indicated satisfaction with the care provided by the chiropractor, with 78.8% of them being very satisfied and 18.9% being satisfied."[6]
- Information on comorbidities is on page 169 of the study "Another important clinical issue in Community Health Centers is the prevalence of serious comorbidities. Most CHC clients had coexisting serious medical or mental health problems. In our two clinics, we had clients who were victims of torture or abuse (past or present) and who had dual diagnoses."[6]
  - *"Patients who have coexisting conditions are more likely to be on multiple drugs in which case adding an analgesic can complicate some coexisting conditions such as GI disorders or heart or stroke concerns. Chiropractic is effective without medication for the management of pain."*
  - The cost-effectiveness data that run alongside this study are also important selling features for this patient demographic; it is discussed in Chapter 10.

Potential Questions and Objections

- There was no control group.
  - *"No, this was a single-group, pre/post intervention study for a frequently overlooked and undertreated patient population. Most patients receiving care in these settings receive care for conditions that could result in death. LBP does not result in death and is therefore not commonly treated. It is now demonstrated that offering care for LBP could improve disability and reduce work absenteeism."*
- Difficult language barriers.
  - A; *"Difficult for every healthcare profession"* (or if you speak a second language you could indicate that as well.)

Patient Types

- Patients who have limited income and coexisting conditions that can complicate their care
- Patients who have a coexisting disability such as a previous heart attack and who should not take NSAIDs. In addition, patients whose pain is

interfering with the ability to work, which literally means the difference between putting food on the table or not.

Bottom Line

"Chiropractic care is effective at treating lower back and neck pain patients with multiple and serious health conditions by decreasing pain, improving disability, and improving overall health status."

"Efficacy of Spinal Manipulation and Mobilization for Low Back Pain and Neck Pain: A Systematic Review and Best Evidence Synthesis." Gert Bronfort, Mitchell Haas, Roni Evans, Lex Bouter. *Spine.* 2004;335–356.

Proof Source

- Systematic review
- Acute, chronic, and mixed lumbar pain efficacy
- Chronic cervical pain
- Safety of lumbar and cervical manipulation
- Head to head of manipulation over GP and PT care for cervical pain and information booklet in mixed lower back pain

Abstract

Background context: Despite the many published randomized clinical trials (RCTs), a substantial number of reviews and several national clinical guidelines, much controversy still remains regarding the evidence for or against efficacy of spinal manipulation for low back pain and neck pain.

Purpose: To reassess the efficacy of spinal manipulative therapy (SMT) and mobilization (MOB) for the management of low back pain (LBP) and neck pain (NP), with special attention to applying more stringent criteria for study admissibility into evidence and for isolating the effect of SMT and/or MOB.

Study design: RCTs including 10 or more subjects per group receiving SMT or MOB and using patient-oriented primary outcome measures (e.g., patient-rated pain, disability, global improvement, and recovery time).

Methods: Articles in English, Danish, Swedish, Norwegian, and Dutch reporting on randomized trials were identified by a comprehensive search of computerized and bibliographic literature databases up to the end of 2002. Two reviewers independently abstracted data and assessed study quality according to eight explicit criteria. A best evidence synthesis incorporating explicit, detailed information about outcome measures and interventions was used to evaluate treatment efficacy. The strength of evidence was assessed by a classification system that incorporated study validity and statistical significance of study results. Sixty-nine RCTs met the study selection criteria and were reviewed and assigned validity scores varying from 6 to 81 on a scale of 0 to 100. Forty-three RCTs met the admissibility criteria for evidence.

Results: *Acute LBP:* There is moderate evidence that SMT provides more short-term pain relief than MOB and detuned diathermy, and limited evidence of faster recovery than a commonly used physical therapy treatment strategy.

Chronic LBP: There is moderate evidence that SMT has an effect similar to an efficacious prescription nonsteroidal anti-inflammatory drug; SMT/MOB is effective in the short term when compared with placebo and general practitioner care, and in the long term compared to physical therapy. There is limited to moderate evidence that SMT is better than physical therapy and home back exercise in both the short and long term. There is limited evidence that SMT is superior to sham SMT in the short term and superior to chemonucleolysis for disc herniation in the short term. However, there is also limited evidence that MOB is inferior to back exercise after disc herniation surgery.

Mix of acute and chronic LBP: SMT/MOB provides either similar or better pain outcomes in the short and long term when compared with placebo and with other treatments, such as McKenzie therapy, medical care, management by physical therapists, soft tissue treatment, and back school.

Acute NP: There are few studies, and the evidence is currently inconclusive.

Chronic NP: There is moderate evidence that SMT/MOB is superior to general practitioner management for short-term pain reduction but that SMT offers at most similar pain relief to high-technology rehabilitative exercise in the short and long term.

Mix of acute and chronic NP: The overall evidence is not clear. There is moderate evidence that MOB is superior to physical therapy and family physician care, and similar to SMT in both the short and long term. There is limited evidence that SMT, in both the short and long term, is inferior to physical therapy.

Conclusions: Our data synthesis suggests that recommendations can be made with some confidence regarding the use of SMT and/or MOB as a viable option for the treatment of both low back pain and NP. There have been few high-quality trials distinguishing between acute and chronic patients, and most are limited to shorter-term follow-up. Future trials should examine well-defined subgroups of patients, further address the value of SMT and MOB for acute patients, establish optimal number of treatment visits, and consider the cost-effectiveness of care.

Promotional Strengths

- Published in *Spine*.
- Published in 2002.
- Variable study populations.
- No adverse events reported (cervical and lumbar).
- Improved methodology over previous systematic or meta-analysis reviews.
- Good for promoting acute and chronic lower back and neck conditions in one study. Head-to-head studies are included so that treatment comparisons are also included in brief format.
- Thirty-one studies for LBP with a total of 5,202 participants met the inclusion criteria.
  - Table 4 on page 340 of the study illustrates the studies that were included for review of acute LBP total 6 studies with $n = 662$. The evidence of efficacy for acute LBP illustrated in the study on page 340, Table 5 includes the following:

    Moderate evidence:
    - ◆ "SMT has better short-term efficacy than spinal mobilization and detuned diathermy."
  - Evidence of efficacy for Chronic LBP (11 trials with $n = 1,472$) is illustrated in Table 6 on page 341 of the study. Table 7 on page 342 of the study summarizes the efficacy:

    Moderate evidence:
    - ◆ "SMT with strengthening exercise is similar in effect to prescription NSAIDs with exercise for pain relief in both the short and long term."
    - ◆ "SMT/MOB is superior to physical therapy and to home exercise for reducing disability in the long term."
    - ◆ "SMT/MOB is superior to general practice medical care and to placebo in the short term, and superior to physical therapy in the long term for patient improvement."
  - Table 8 on pages 343 and 344 of the study lists the evidence of efficacy for a mix of acute and chronic lower back pain (14 trials with $n = 3,068$).

    Table 9 on page 344 of the study illustrates the evidence of efficacy for moderate evidence:
    - ◆ "SMT is superior to an information booklet for pain reduction in the short term, but similar in the long term."

- ◆ "In the short and long term, SMT is similar to the following for pain and disability:

    McKenzie therapy, medical care with exercise instruction, soft tissue therapy, physical therapy, and back school."

    "SMT is similar to medical care in the short term."
- Table 14 on page 347 of the study illustrates the five studies included with $n = 444$ participants that were investigated for chronic neck pain.
    - Table 15 on page 347 of the study illustrates the evidence of efficacy for chronic cervical pain:

        Moderate evidence:

        - ◆ "SMT/MOB is superior to general practice medical care and PT in the short term for improving functioning."
        - ◆ "SMT is at most similar to high-technology rehabilitative exercise in the short term and long term."
        - ◆ "SMT/MOB is similar in effect to detuned modalities in the short term."
    - Table 16 on page 348 of the study illustrates the five trials that were included, with $n = 638$ and that were investigated for a mix of acute and chronic neck pain:

        Table 17 on page 348 of the study illustrates the evidence of efficacy for a mix of acute and chronic neck pain.

        - ◆ "Moderate evidence:

            MOB is superior to PT for pain control in the short and long term and superior to medical care in the short term.

            SMT and MOB are similar in the short and long term."
- Page 346 of the study indicates that "There are now more randomized controlled clinical trials on spinal manipulation for the management of LBP than for any other treatment method."[7]
- Side effects and complications from manipulation are discussed on page 351 of the study.
    - "The risk of irreversible cauda equina syndrome is estimated to be as low as 1 in 100 million lumbar spine manipulations."[7]
    - "There are currently 46 RCTs published on spinal manipulation for LBP involving over 5,000 patients. No serious adverse events have been reported in these trials."[7]
    - "Individual estimates and the results of the retrospective surveys consistently suggest a risk of serious cerebrovascular complication of approximately 1 per 1 million cervical manipulations."[7]

- Cost-effectiveness information can be found on page 352 of the study:
  - "The most comprehensive cost-effectiveness analysis to date was performed by Hoving et al. The trial compared MOB, physical therapy and general practitioner care for a case mix of acute and chronic NP. MOB was more cost effective than the other two interventions both in the short and long term."[7]

Potential Questions and Objections

- There are no graphs that pop out and make a verbal presentation easy to explain with visual aids.
  - The reason this study is important is primarily because it is a good overall study that provides an overview of the efficacy of manipulation for lower back and cervical treatments. It also offers another systematic review to overcome the Cochrane Back Review Summary discussed in Chapter 5.
- Some of the treatment methods discussed are now obsolete.
  - True, but there are many other studies to turn to based on the doctor's interest.

Patient Types

- A patient type is not necessarily appropriate for this study. Rather, this study is appropriate for a doctor requesting a systematic review of manipulation.

Bottom Line

"Manipulation and mobilization by chiropractors can be confidently recommended as viable options for the treatment of both low back and neck pain."

The next three studies on chronic spinal pain syndromes are all related, and each one is a continuation of the previous one. These studies compare short-term and long-term data for chronic spinal pain syndromes using acupuncture, NSAIDs, and SMT. The first study, which was published in 1999, gives some background information not available in the final study and which will aid in a full and complete understanding of the methodology. The 2003 *Spine* study is a solid proof source for the rare doctor who objects to a chiropractic journal or for a doctor who you know values research published in that journal. The 2005 *JMPT* study is the most recent and has the long-term data, making it the top choice of the three for promoting. Keep in mind that due to the small study size, these are not the best choice for a first meeting with a physician.

"Chronic Spinal Pain Syndromes: A Clinical Pilot Trial Comparing Acupuncture, a Nonsteroidal Anti-inflammatory Drug, and Spinal Manipulation." Lynton G. F. Giles and Reinhold Müller. *Journal of Manipulative and Physiological Therapeutics.* 1999;22:376–381.

Proof Source

- Manipulation is more efficacious than acupuncture and NSAIDs for chronic lower back and neck pain.
- Efficacy of manipulation in pain and disability for chronic lower back and neck pain
- Side effects of medication
- Discharge (recovery) rates highest for manipulation

Abstract

Objective: To compare needle acupuncture, medication (tenoxicam with ranitidine), and spinal manipulation for managing chronic (> 13 weeks' duration) spinal pain syndromes.

Design: Prospective, randomized, independently assessed preintervention and postintervention clinical pilot trial.

Setting: Specialized spinal pain syndrome outpatient unit at Townsville General Hospital, Queensland, Australia.

Subjects: Seventy-seven patients (without contraindication to manipulation or medication) were recruited.

Interventions: One of three separate, clearly defined intervention protocols: needle acupuncture, nonsteroidal anti-inflammatory medication, or chiropractic spinal manipulation.

Main Outcome Measures: Main outcome measures were changes (4 weeks vs initial visit) in the scores of the (1) Oswestry Back Pain Disability Index, (2) Neck Disability Index, and (3) three visual analogue scales of local pain intensity.

Results: Randomization was successful. After a median intervention period of 30 days, spinal manipulation was the only intervention that achieved statistically significant improvements (all expressed as percentages of the original scores) with (1) a reduction of 30.7% on the Oswestry scale, (2) an improvement of 25% on the neck disability index, and (3) reductions on the visual analogue scale of 50% for low back pain, 46% for upper back pain, and 33% for neck pain (all $P < 0.001$). Neither of the other interventions showed any significant improvement on any of the outcome measures.

Conclusions: The consistency of the results provides, in spite of several discussed shortcomings of this pilot study, evidence that in patients with chronic spinal pain syndromes spinal manipulation, if not contraindicated, results in greater improvement than acupuncture and medicine.

Promotional Strengths

- Published in *JMPT.*
- Despite small $n = 77$, the findings were "consistently statistically significant for the manipulation group only in every outcome measure." The strength of this outcome helps overcome the small study size.
- "The only side effects including serious adverse events were gastric symptoms in the medication group." (p. 379)
- Head-to-head data illustrating manipulation as more efficacious than medication and acupuncture for chronic spinal pain.
- Familiar outcome measures: VAS, Oswestry Disability score, NDI.
- "Of the 19 patients discharged, 39% were in the manipulation group, 10% in the acupuncture group, 14.3% in the medication group." (p. 379)
- Table 1 on page 378 of the study illustrates: "Patients had pain for at least 13 weeks and the average disability was moderate with the majority of patients being male."
- Table 2A on page 379 of the study provides strong and compelling data for manipulation over acupuncture and medication. "The manipulation group demonstrated a robust statistical significance for efficacy based on the Oswestry Disability rating for lumbar pain over acupuncture and medication."
- Table 2B on page 379 of the study provides strong and compelling data for manipulation over acupuncture and medication. "The only group to demonstrate statistical significance was the manipulation

group for efficacy based on the Neck Disability Index rating for cervical pain."

- Table 3A on page 380 of the study provides strong and compelling data for manipulation over acupuncture and medication. "The only group to demonstrate statistical significance was the manipulation group for efficacy based on the Visual Analog Scale for the lower back."

- Table 3B on page 380 of the study provides strong and compelling data for manipulation over acupuncture and medication. "The manipulation group again demonstrates robust statistical significance for pain related to the upper back based on the Visual Analog Scale."

- Table 3C on page 380 of the study provides strong and compelling data for manipulation over acupuncture and medication. "The manipulation group again demonstrates robust statistical significance for pain related to the neck based on the Visual Analog Scale."

Potential Questions and Objections

- The doctor may not recognize the medication that is listed.
  - "The NSAID used is not available in the United States, but it is widely used in Australia. Specifically, the patients took tenoxicam with ranitidine. In the United States, ranitidine, as you know, has a brand name of Zantac, which is used for heartburn and is a H_2 antagonist. Although it isn't a drug used here in the United States, it is in the NSAID class. Does that alleviate any concern you have with the medication arm of this study?" If it does not, move to another study with NSAID usage."
  - NSAIDs are a huge class of drugs, all of which are considered to be efficacious. The point here is that manipulation produced statistically significant results over the medication and is safer than medication with fewer side effects.
- The abstract mentions shortcomings in this study. What are they?
  - "The study site was in tropical Australia. The next major medical community was 1,250 kilometers, or 750 miles, away. This created logistical problems with patient follow-up and for the acupuncture group difficulty obtaining appointments, which prolonged the time to apply the treatments. Finally, funding restrictions resulted in understaffing, which resulted in randomization to be stopped prior to all envelopes being used. The results of the study are impressive and robust, despite the size of study participants and shortcomings."

- The study size seems small.
  - "Due to the strictness of the inclusion and exclusion criteria, 875 patients were considered for the study, and 745 were excluded. This underscores the homogenous nature of the study participants and lends greater credibility to the results. In addition, statistical testing takes the sample size into consideration."

Patient Types

- For patients who have chronic pain with motion, neck stiffness, and who wake up with pain, NSAIDs are usually a first choice; however, patients who are at risk of heart disease or stroke have their risk increase when taking NSAIDs. Manipulation is the best and safest alternative.
- For patients who have coexisting stomach disorders that could be exacerbated by NSAIDs, manipulation is a less invasive and more efficacious treatment choice.
- For patients who are trying to choose a noninvasive form of treatment, manipulation was found to be more efficacious than acupuncture for chronic lower back and neck pain.

Bottom Line

"Patients with chronic pain had consistent statistically significant improvements above acupuncture and medication without the side effects or safety warnings of NSAIDs."

"Chronic Spinal Pain: A Randomized Clinical Trial Comparing Medication, Acupuncture, and Spinal Manipulation." L.G. Giles and R. Muller. *Spine.* 2003;28(14):1490–1502.

Proof Source

- Manipulation is more efficacious than acupuncture and NSAIDs for chronic lower back and neck pain.
- Efficacy of manipulation in pain and disability for chronic lower back and neck pain
- Side effects of medication
- Discharge (recovery) rates highest for manipulation

Abstract

Study design: A randomized controlled clinical trial was conducted.

Objective: To compare medication, needle acupuncture, and spinal manipulation for managing chronic (> 13 weeks' duration) spinal pain because the value of medicinal and popular forms of alternative care for chronic spinal pain syndromes is uncertain.

Summary of background data: Between February 1999 and October 2001, 115 patients without contraindication for the three treatment regimens were enrolled at the public hospital's multidisciplinary spinal pain unit.

Methods: One of three separate intervention protocols was used: medication, needle acupuncture, or chiropractic spinal manipulation. Patients were assessed before treatment by a sports medical physician for exclusion criteria and by a research assistant using the Oswestry Back Pain Disability Index (Oswestry), the Neck Disability Index (NDI), the Short-Form-36 Health Survey questionnaire (SF-36), visual analog scales (VAS) of pain intensity and ranges of movement. These instruments were administered again at 2, 5, and 9 weeks after the beginning of treatment.

Results: Randomization proved to be successful. The highest proportion of early (asymptomatic status) recovery was found for manipulation (27.3%), followed by acupuncture (9.4%) and medication (5%). Manipulation achieved the best overall results, with improvements of 50% ($P = 0.01$) on the Oswestry scale, 38% ($P = 0.08$) on the NDI, 47% ($P < 0.001$) on the SF-36, and 50% ($P < 0.01$) on the VAS for back pain, 38% ($P < 0.001$) for lumbar standing flexion, 20% ($P < 0.001$) for lumbar sitting flexion, 25% ($P = 0.1$) for cervical sitting flexion, and 18% ($P = 0.02$) for cervical sitting extension. However, on the VAS for neck pain, acupuncture showed a better result than manipulation (50% vs 42%).

Conclusions: The consistency of the results provides, despite some discussed shortcomings of this study, evidence that in patients with chronic spinal pain, manipulation, if not contraindicated, results in greater short-term improvement than acupuncture or medication. However, the data do not strongly support the use of only manipulation, only acupuncture, or only nonsteroidal anti-inflammatory drugs for the treatment of chronic spinal pain. The results from this exploratory study need confirmation from future larger studies.

Promotional Strengths

- Published in *Spine.*
- Recent publication date of 2003.
- Adverse events (cervical and lumbar).

- Longer follow-up from the original study.
- Familiar outcome measures: VAS, Oswestry Disability Score, NDI.
- All other promotional strengths for the original study remain and, with the exception of one, continued to improve:
  - Original findings in *JMPT* 1999 study as discussed earlier and expanded upon in this study indicated that "manipulation was responsible for the following outcome improvement rates:"
    - ➤ "Oswestry: 30.7%; NDI: 25%; VAS low back: 50%; VAS neck pain: 33%."
  - "Findings in the 9-week follow-up showed increased improvements as follows:"
    - ➤ "Oswestry: 50%; NDI: 47%; VAS LB: 50%; VAS neck pain: 42% for manipulation; however, acupuncture had 50%."
- With regards to achieving an asymptomatic status:
  - *JMPT* 1999 study
    - ➤ Manipulation 39%; Acupuncture 10%; Medication 14.3%
  - Nine-week follow-up study
    - ➤ "Manipulation 27.3%; Acupuncture 9.4%; Medication 5%"
  - "This reflects the fact that patients who respond to manipulation stay better, whereas with medication the response is short lived."

Potential Questions and Objections

- The same weaknesses apply as in the original study.
- Presuming you have membership access to *JMPT* and do not subscribe to *Spine*, the cost of providing the *Spine* study is more expensive for promotion. However, if a doctor does not like *JMPT*, it is convenient to have this study that was published in *Spine* as an alternate proof source of the same material.

Patient Types

- For a patient who has chronic pain with motion, neck stiffness, and who wakes up with pain, NSAIDs use is the first choice; however, patients who are at risk of heart disease or stroke have their risk increase when taking NSAIDs. Manipulation is the best and safest alternative.
- For patients who have coexisting stomach disorders that could be exacerbated by NSAIDs, manipulation is a less invasive and more efficacious treatment choice.

- For patients who are trying to choose a noninvasive form of treatment, manipulation was found to be more efficacious than acupuncture for chronic lower back and neck pain.

Bottom Line

"Patients with chronic pain had consistent statistically significant improvements above acupuncture and medication without the side effects or safety warnings of NSAIDs. When these patients were followed after the initial study period, it was found that patients who had manipulation retained their efficacy."

"Long-Term Follow-Up of a Randomized Clinical Trial Assessing the Efficacy of Medication, Acupuncture, and Spinal Manipulation for Chronic Mechanical Spinal Pain Syndromes." Reinhold Muller and Lynton G.F. Giles. *Journal of Manipulative and Physiological Therapeutics.* 2005;28:3–11.

Proof Source

- Significant efficacy for chiropractic manipulation for the short- and long-term benefit of chronic neck and lower back pain
- Manipulation is more efficacious than acupuncture and NSAIDs for chronic neck and lower back pain.
- Efficacy of manipulation in pain and disability for chronic neck and lower back pain
- Side effects of medication
- Discharge (recovery) rates highest for manipulation

Abstract

Objective: To assess the long-term benefits of medication, needle acupuncture and spinal manipulation as exclusive and standardized treatment regimens in patients with chronic (13 weeks) spinal pain syndromes.

Study design: Extended follow-up (1 year) of a randomized clinical trial was conducted at the multidisciplinary spinal pain unit of Townsville's General Hospital between February 1999 and October 2001.

Patients and methods: Of the 115 patients originally randomized, 69 had exclusively been treated with the randomly allocated treatment during the 9-week treatment period (results at 9 weeks were reported earlier). These patients were followed up and assessed again 1 year after inception into the study by reapplying the same instruments (ie, Oswestry Back Pain Index, Neck Disability Index, Short-Form-36, and Visual Analogue Scales). Questionnaires were obtained from 62 patients reflecting a retention proportion of 90%. The main analysis was restricted to 40 patients who had received exclusively the randomly allocated treatment for the whole observation period since randomization.

Results: Comparisons of initial and extended follow-up questionnaires to assess absolute efficacy showed that only the application of spinal manipulation revealed broad-based long-term benefit: 5 of the 7 main outcome measures showed significant improvements compared with only 1 item in each of the acupuncture and the medication groups.

Conclusions: In patients with chronic spinal pain syndromes, spinal manipulation, if not contraindicated, may be the only treatment modality of the assessed regimens that provides broad and significant long-term benefit.

Promotional Strengths

- Published in *JMPT.*
- Recent publication date: 2005.
- No adverse events occurred.
- Head-to-head data and 1-year follow-up of an RCT.
- Despite small $n = 62$, the findings were consistently statistically significant for the manipulation-only group in every outcome measure.
- Familiar outcome measures: VAS, Oswestry Disability Score, NDI.
- The only side effects were in the medication group, which included Celebrex, Vioxx, and acetaminophen.
- Table 2 on page 7 of the study examines all of the outcome scores: "In this updated study, the long-term values were in favor of manipulation, improved for acupuncture, and some deterioration was noted in the medication arm."
- Table 3 on page 8 of the study illustrates "that five of seven of the outcome scores showed statistical significance from the original assessment to the extended assessment in manipulation, one in acupuncture,

and one in medication." (It is helpful to highlight the statistically significant *p* values in all treatment groups of Table 3 to visually add impact to the findings.)

- "Patients who had to change their treatment because of no response or side effects were highest in the medication group and lowest in the manipulation group."

Potential Questions and Objections

- When did patients change their treatment?
  - "Patients were allowed to change at any time after randomization, which is similar to what you would do with patients in your own office if they were not responding to your first choice of treatment."

The study population is small.

  - "It is smaller than other studies, but it is the only head-to-head data available directly comparing acupuncture, medication, and manipulation in the same study. As such, because of the smaller sample size, the outcomes need to stand out as superior. The fact that only manipulation showed significant improvements in this long-term data in five out of seven outcomes and acupuncture and medication showed significant improvements in one out of seven outcomes each is compelling evidence. In addition, the study and findings were compelling enough and important enough to be published on three separate occasions in *Spine* and *JMPT*."

Patient Types

- For a patient who has chronic pain with motion, neck stiffness, and who wakes up with pain, NSAIDs may be first choice; however, patients who are at risk of heart disease or stroke have their risk increase when taking NSAIDs. Manipulation is the best and safest alternative.
- For patients who have coexisting stomach disorders that could be exacerbated by NSAIDs, manipulation is a less invasive and more efficacious treatment choice.
- For patients who are trying to choose a noninvasive form of treatment, manipulation was found to be more efficacious than acupuncture for chronic lower back and neck pain.
- For patients who have had previous treatment failures, manipulation has proven to be efficacious in both the short and long term over NSAIDs and acupuncture.

Bottom Line

> *"Patients with chronic back pain do well with manipulation and exhibit consistent statistically significant improvements over medication and acupuncture one year after the study."*

Section IV: Headache Studies

The studies included in this section are primarily headache oriented; however, many studies in the section titled "Section II: Cervical Studies" earlier in this chapter provide patient demographics with headaches listed as one of the common symptoms. As such, referring to those studies to examine the outcome of manipulation on headaches related to cervical pain is also appropriate to demonstrate the efficacy of manual therapies for the treatment of headaches.

"Efficacy of Spinal Manipulation for Chronic Headache: A Systematic Review." Gert Bronfort, Willem J.J. Assendelft, Roni Evans, Mitchell Haas, and Lex Bouter. *Journal of Manipulative and Physiological Therapeutics.* 2001;24:457–466.

Proof Source

- Efficacy of manipulation for migraine, tension, and cervicogenic headaches
- Efficacy and safety of manipulation over medication, which aids in treatment compliance

Abstract

Background: Chronic headache is a prevalent condition with substantial socioeconomic impact. Complementary or alternative therapies are increasingly being used by patients to treat headache pain, and spinal manipulative therapy (SMT) is among the most common of these.

Objective: To assess the efficacy/effectiveness of SMT for chronic headache through a systematic review of randomized clinical trials.

Study selection: Randomized clinical trials on chronic headache (tension, migraine, and cervicogenic) were included in the review if they compared SMT with other interventions or placebo. The trials had to have at least 1 patient-rated outcome measure such as pain severity, frequency, duration, improvement, use of analgesics, disability, or quality of life. Studies were identified through a comprehensive search of MEDLINE (1966–1998) and EMBASE (1974–1998). Additionally, all available data from the Cumulative Index of Nursing and Allied Health Literature, the Chiropractic Research Archives Collection, and the Manual, Alternative, and Natural Therapies Information System were used, as well as material gathered through the citation tracking, and hand searching of nonindexed chiropractic, osteopathic, and manual medicine journals.

Data extraction: Information about outcome measures, interventions, and effect sizes was used to evaluate treatment efficacy. Levels of evidence were determined by a classification system incorporating study validity and statistical significance of study results. Two authors independently extracted data and performed methodological scoring of selected trials.

Data synthesis: Nine trials involving 683 patients with chronic headache were included. The methodological quality (validity) scores ranged from 21 to 87 (100-point scale). The trials were too heterogeneous in terms of patient clinical characteristics, control groups, and outcome measures to warrant statistical pooling. Based on predefined criteria, there is moderate evidence that SMT has short-term efficacy similar to amitriptyline in the prophylactic treatment of chronic tension-type headache and migraine. SMT does not appear to improve outcomes when added to soft-tissue massage for episodic tension-type headache. There is moderate evidence that SMT is more efficacious than massage for cervicogenic headache. Sensitivity analyses showed that the results and the overall study conclusions remained the same even when substantial changes in the prespecified assumptions/rules regarding the evidence determination were applied.

Conclusions: SMT appears to have a better effect than massage for cervicogenic headache. It also appears that SMT has an effect comparable to commonly used first-line prophylactic prescription medications for tension-type headache and migraine headache. This conclusion rests upon a few trials of adequate methodological quality. Before any firm conclusions can be drawn, further testing should be done in rigorously designed, executed, and analyzed trials with follow-up periods of sufficient length.

Promotional Strengths

- Published in *JMPT.*
- Authors are prominent thought leaders in the chiropractic industry.

- Large study population: $n = 683$.
- Systematic review.
- Table 2 on page 460 of the study provides an overview of the studies that were examined. They are listed by methodological score. It is a good table to initiate a conversation focused on the different types of headaches that could be treated by manipulation and a quick glimpse of the comparator treatment and outcome.
- Figure 1 on page 461 of the study is a nice visual aid for discussing several studies with strong validity scores that favored spinal manipulation:
  - "More trials favored spinal manipulation than those that didn't. In fact, only one trial did not favor manipulation in its entirety and stands out as the exception rather than the rule."
- Side effects and safety are noted on page 462 of the study.
  - "In the studies comparing SMT with amitriptyline, more than half the patients taking amitriptyline reported side effects such as drowsiness, dry mouth, and weight gain, and approximately 10% were withdrawn from the studies due to drug intolerance. In comparison, only 5% of the patients receiving SMT reported side effects, the most frequent being muscle soreness and neck stiffness. These effects are common and considered normal reactions to spinal manipulation."[8]
  - "No serious complications (that is, vertebrobasilar accidents) were reported in any of the studies included in this review. The risk of serious complications from SMT is considered low."[8]

Potential Questions and Objections

- The study is older and newer studies may be more appropriate. However, it is one of the most recent *systematic* reviews, which is why it was included in this text.
- The authors discuss a valid point that many of the included studies have low methodological quality and medication withdrawal, which is not consistent with common medical practice. In other words, if you introduce a study that illustrates a finding that conflicts with common medical experience, the study loses credibility or at the very least fails to make an impression on the doctor.
  - Agree that you understand that this is not a common finding, but use the statement to discuss the safety and low side effects of manipulation compared to medication. "Patient care is compromised if side effects from medication prevent them from being compliant."

Patient Types

- Patients with chronic headaches that inhibit their ability to work or activities of daily living
- Patients not compliant to medication or experiencing unpleasant side effects

Bottom Line

"Manipulation consistently provides relief from pain and decreases reliance on medication for patients with migraines, tension and cervicogenic headaches, and it is proven to be safe and associated with high compliance with treatment."

"Evidence Report: Behavioral and Physical Treatments for Tension-Type and Cervicogenic Headache: Duke University Evidence-Based Practice Center." Douglas C. McCrory, Donald B. Penzien, Vic Hasselblad, Rebecca N. Gray. Des Moines, IA: Foundation for Chiropractic Education and Research; 2001.

Proof Source

- Efficacy data for the treatment of headaches including manipulation, physiotherapy, behavioral therapy, acupuncture, soft tissue massage, and medication

Abstract

Objectives: To identify and summarize evidence from controlled trials on the efficacy of behavioral and physical treatments for tension-type and cervicogenic headache.

Search strategy: A strategy combining the MeSH term *headache* (exploded) and a previously published strategy for identifying randomized controlled trials was used on the January 1966 to December 1999 MEDLINE database. Other computerized bibliographical databases, textbooks, and experts were also utilized.

Selection criteria: English-language controlled trials involving patients with tension-type or cervicogenic headache in which at least one treatment offered was a behavioral or physical treatment were selected.

Data collection and analysis: Measures of headache index and headache frequency reported as group means (and standard deviations) were used to calculate standardized mean differences (or effect sizes). Where similar trials provided data, meta-analysis of efficacy measures was performed. The number of patients obtaining at least a 50% reduction in headache index, frequency, or severity was recorded and used to calculate odds ratios.

Main results: Behavioral treatments for tension-type headache have a consistent body of research indicating efficacy. Summary effect sizes from a meta-analysis of 23 trials suggest that relaxation training, cognitive-behavioral therapy, electromyographic (EMG) biofeedback combined with relaxation training, and EMG biofeedback without relaxation training were all effective in treating tension-type headache when compared to a wait-list control. In addition, these behavioral treatments were similar in effectiveness to drug treatment with amitriptyline. Physical treatments have been less often studied. Six small trials of acupuncture yielded inconsistent results. Cervical spinal manipulation effectively relieved headaches compared with control treatments in two studies of patients with headache and neck pain and/or neck dysfunction, but its effectiveness in patients with tension-type headache is less clear, since no placebo or no-treatment control studies of manipulation have been performed in this population. One trial conducted among patients with tension-type headache showed that manipulation conferred no extra benefit when added to soft-tissue therapy. In another trial conducted among patients with tension-type headache, manipulation was less effective than amitriptyline at reducing headache intensity after 6 weeks of treatment; unlike amitriptyline, however, manipulation provided a sustained response for up to 4 weeks after cessation of treatment. Other physical treatments for which controlled trials have been reported include cranial electrical stimulation, aerobic exercise, and therapeutic touch.

Conclusions: Each of the behavioral therapies considered has modest efficacy for tension-type headache. There is little information about which patients will benefit from particular behavioural approaches; the choice among them may, for the present, depend more on availability and acceptability than on data about efficacy. Manipulation is effective in patients with cervicogenic headaches, but its efficacy in patients with tension-type headache is unproven. There are insufficient data about any of the other physical treatments to draw conclusions about their efficacy.

Promotional Strengths

- Conducted by Duke University, which has been awarded the trade-marked designation of "EPC" (Evidence-based Practice Center) by the Agency for Healthcare Research and Quality.
- Conducted by 19 multidisciplinary doctors.
- Promotes and identifies appropriate treatments based on the literature.
- Contains competitor studies such as acupuncture where no strong findings were identified for the efficacy of acupuncture in treating tension-type and cervicogenic headaches. In addition, it examined head-to-head studies against physiotherapy and medication. This is discussed in more detail in Chapter 11.
- Thorough account on all treatment options for tension-type and cervicogenic headaches. Offering a product manuscript on headaches is appropriate and is best used for a doctor who is interested in the treatment of headaches.
- Evidence in Table 2 on page 146 of the report lists several studies that can be used and highlighted for doctors:
  - Page 146 outlines a study done by Boline et al. in 1995:
    Spinal manipulation vs. amitriptyline for the treatment of chronic tension-type headaches: a randomized clinical trial. *J Manipulative Physiol Ther.* 1995;18(3):148–154.
    - Study population: $n = 150$
    - Short trial of manipulation with proven efficacy
    - Side effects that caused dropouts in the medication group. (If doctor indicates dosage was not appropriate, it could be because the patient couldn't tolerate the medication. In addition, while they have to titrate up the medication, manipulation patients are gaining full therapeutic effects immediately, reducing the time needed to see improvements.)
- Page 148 of the report outlines a study by G. Bove and N. Nilsson.
  - Spinal manipulation in the treatment of episodic tension-type headache: a randomized controlled trial. *JAMA.* 1998;280(18):1576–1579.
    Study population: $n = 75$
    Treatment groups SMT and massage versus massage + laser light therapy
    Both groups had significant reduction in headache duration
    Both groups maintained their effects for the remaining trial

This trial illustrates the importance of a placebo and control group. The treatment effect of SMT is difficult to isolate.

- Page 159 of the report outlines a study by Nilsson, Christensen, and Hartvigsen in 1997:
  - The effect of spinal manipulation in the treatment of cervicogenic headache. *J Manipulative Physiol Ther.* 1997;20(5):326–330.

    Study population: $n = 53$

    SMT versus soft tissue therapy

    Headache frequency, duration, and severity were significantly reduced from week 1 to week 5 with manipulation.

Note: Of the six studies utilized in the Duke report, it is best to focus on the ones listed here. The others were not outlined either because of the publication date, size of sample, conclusions, or inability to determine who conducted the adjustments.

Potential Questions or Objections:

- Several trials are older (1979, 1983, 1990, 1995).
- Most trials lack a control or placebo.
- Some trials included in review had small n.
- Lacks graphs and charts for visual detailing.
- Not all trials were conclusive for manipulation; however, this is easily refuted based on sample size and the fact that SMT was not always isolated as a treatment.
- The publication date of 2001 makes it an older report; however, because of its in-depth coverage, it is still a valuable promotional source and frequently referred to in the literature.

Patient Types

- Patients with tension or cervicogenic headaches

Bottom Line

"Cervical spine manipulation was associated with significant improvement in headache outcome involving patients with neck pain and/or neck dysfunction and headache."

"A Randomized Controlled Trial of Chiropractic Spinal Manipulative Therapy for Migraine." Peter J. Tuchin, Henry Pollard, and Rod Bonello. *Journal of Manipulative and Physiological Therapeutics.* 2000;23:91–95.

Proof Source

- Efficacy for manipulation in migraine headaches
- Safety (cervical)

Abstract

Objective: To assess the efficacy of chiropractic spinal manipulative therapy (SMT) in the treatment of migraine.

Design: A randomized controlled trial of 6 months' duration. The trial consisted of 3 stages: 2 months of data collection (before treatment), 2 months of treatment, and a further 2 months of data collection (after treatment). Comparison of outcomes to the initial baseline factors was made at the end of the 6 months for both an SMT group and a control group.

Setting: Chiropractic Research Center of Macquarie University.

Participants: One hundred twenty-seven volunteers between the ages of 10 and 70 years were recruited through media advertising. The diagnosis of migraine was made on the basis of the International Headache Society standard, with a minimum of at least one migraine per month.

Interventions: Two months of chiropractic SMT (diversified technique) at vertebral fixations determined by the practitioner (maximum of 16 treatments).

Main outcome measures: Participants completed standard headache diaries during the entire trial noting the frequency, intensity (visual analogue score), duration, disability, associated symptoms, and use of medication for each migraine episode.

Results: The average response of the treatment group ($n = 83$) showed statistically significant improvement in migraine frequency ($P < 0.005$), duration ($P < 0.01$), disability ($P < 0.05$), and medication use ($P < 0.001$) when compared with the control group ($n = 40$). Four persons failed to complete the trial because of a variety of causes, including change in residence, a motor vehicle accident, and increased migraine frequency. Expressed in other terms, 22% of participants reported more than a 90% reduction of migraines as a consequence of the 2 months of SMT. Approximately 50% more participants reported significant improvement in the morbidity of each episode.

Conclusions: The results of this study support previous results showing that some people report significant improvement in migraines after chiropractic SMT. A high percentage (> 80%) of participants reported stress as a major factor for their migraines. It appears probable that chiropractic care has an effect on the physical conditions related to stress and that in these people the effects of the migraine are reduced.

Promotional Strengths

- Published in *JMPT.*
- Randomized controlled trial.
- Discusses etiology of migraines and how manipulation may play an effective role in treatment.
- Patients kept a headache diary 2 months prior to treatment, 2 months during the treatment, and 2 months after the treatment, which provides a nice summary on the effect of treatment.
- Table 1 on page 93 of the study illustrates: "Patients had an average of 7 migraines a month that lasted on average 22 to 23 hours and caused disability for approximately 19 hours of the 22 to 23 hours. On average patients had an 18-year history of migraines."
- Table 2 on page 93 of the study illustrates common symptoms associated with migraines that are extremely useful to build a patient type such as photophobia and nausea.
- Figures 1, 2, 3, and 4 on pages 93 and 94 of the study provide visual aids that illustrate the decline in frequency, disability hours, and duration hours for the manipulation group. All but Figure 2 on page 93 of the study (VAS) represent a statistically significant decline. "Migraine patients treated with manipulation had statistically significant reductions in disability hours and duration of migraines."
- Table 3 on page 95 of the study: "A statistical significance in overall use in medication, which declined from 21 pills to 10 pills per month, was observed in the manipulation group and a significant number of patients' medication usage had reduced to zero by the end of the trial (page 94 column 1, paragraph 1)."

Potential Questions and Objections

- Medical doctors may not understand some of the "chiropractic" terminology discussed in the methodology section.
  - Instead describe it. For instance vertebral subluxation could be explained as hypomobility.
- Small study population: $n = 127$.
  - Yes, but wouldn't you agree that any chronic migraine patient would be receptive to any therapy that showed a potential decrease in disability and duration of a migraine?
- Although the study is 6 months long, it only examined the effect of treatment for 2 months after the conclusion of treatment.
  - "Decreasing a patient's medication by more than half is significant. It may not be a cure, but affecting the quality of life of a patient who has suffered for 18 years, as many patients in this study had, is also significant and provides a safer and less invasive treatment."

Patient Types

- Patient with headaches who present with symptoms such as one-sided, pulsing of moderate to severe intensity such that they are required to seek a dark or quiet room. Additionally, the patient may have nausea and vomiting and increased pain with neck movement.

Bottom Line

"Patients with migraines and associated photophobia and nausea can have significant relief in terms of disability and frequency resulting in decreased utilization of medication and improved quality of life."

REFERENCES

1. Coudeyre E, Tubach F, Rannou F, et al. Effect of a simple information booklet on pain persistence after an acute episode of low back pain: a non-randomized trial in a primary care setting. *PLoS ONE*. 2(8):e706.
2. Chou R, Qaseem A, Snow V, et al. Diagnosis and treatment of low back pain: a joint clinical practice guideline from the American College of Physicians and the American Pain Society. *Ann Intern Med*. 2007;147:478–491.

3. UK Back pain Exercise and Manipulation (UK BEAM) Trial Team. UK Back pain Exercise And Manipulation (UK BEAM) trial—national randomized trial of physical treatments for back pain in primary care: objectives, design and interventions. *BMC Health Services Research*. 2003;3:13. Available at http://www.biomedcentral.com/1472-6963/3/16.

4. Haas M, Goldberg B, Aickin M, Ganger B, Attwood M. A practice-based study of patients with acute and chronic low back pain attending primary care and chiropractic physicians: two-week to 48-month follow-up. *J Manipulative Physiol Ther*. 2004; 27:160–169.

5. Hoving J, Koes B, de Vet H, et al. Manual therapy, physical therapy, or continued care by a general practitioner for patients with neck pain; a randomized, controlled trial. *Ann Intern Med*. 2002;136:713–722.

6. Garner M, Aker P, Balon J, et al. Chiropractic care of musculoskeletal disorders in a unique population within Canadian community health centers. *J Manipulative Physiol Ther*. 2007;30:165–170.

7. Bronfort G, Haas M, Evans R, Bouter L. Efficacy of spinal manipulation and mobilization for low back pain and neck pain: a systematic review and best evidence synthesis. *Spine*. 2004;335–356.

8. Bronfort G, Assendelft W, Evans R, Haas M, Bouter L. Efficacy of spinal manipulation for chronic headache: a systematic review. *J Manipulative Physiol Ther*. 2001; 24:457–466.

Chapter 9

Safety Data
for Chiropractic

"Guilty Until Proven Innocent"

The safety of manipulation, especially that of the cervical spine, is often misunderstood. It is a fact that a risk exists, but it is minimal especially when the risk is compared to other standard and accepted interventions for treating the spine such as nonsteroidal anti-inflammatory drugs (NSAIDs) and surgery. NSAIDs alone are responsible for more than 16,000 deaths and 100,000 hospitalizations each year, according to the Food and Drug Administration, yet the medical world is fine with prescribing them on a routine basis when not contraindicated and accepts the risk because of the benefit to the patient. In contrast, NCMIC, one of the largest malpractice insurance companies, estimated that for 24,000 insured chiropractors the risk rate for a serious complication following cervical manipulation is approximately 1 in 2 million procedures, or 1 case for each 25 practitioners who all practice for a 40-year period.[1]

Your objective when illustrating the safety of manipulation to a physician is not to be on an anti-medication, anti-physical therapy, or anti-surgery crusade. Rather, it is to educate the doctor that the benefits outweigh the risks for manipulation, and that when it comes to risks of manipulation compared to other treatment protocols, it is far safer without compromising the benefits. In fact, the efficacy of manipulation as illustrated in Chapter 8 is oftentimes superior to the comparator treatment, both in efficacy as well as safety.

Many medical doctors are unaware that chiropractors practice evidence-based medicine. In addition, many simply don't know what a chiropractic visit consists of. Many doctors will be surprised to learn that chiropractors actually conduct orthopedic and neurological testing. They will be further surprised and therefore impressed that not only do chiropractors understand these tests, but they also understand the importance of prescreening patients for cardiovascular risks as well as continual monitoring of adverse side effects. Aside from the research presented in this chapter, your exam and initial health intake forms will bring credibility to your skills and knowledge and to the competent treatment that you deliver to the patient.

There is no doubt that the literature both in scientific journals as well as news periodicals has reported on the more rare and serious complications of manipulation. Some reports may in fact be accurate because there is a risk with manipulation, no matter how minimal it is. It is not 100% safe even for the most careful and competent chiropractor; however, the research illustrates in this chapter the overall risk profile of cervical manipulation is minimal.

There are a few opponents in the medical community to manipulation. It doesn't matter that they exist; what does matter is the validity of their studies and conclusions on which they base their negative opinions. If a medical doctor presents a negative study on manipulation (it is unlikely that a negative study on the adverse events of manipulation could possibly be worse than the adverse events of NSAIDs!), take the following considerations into account:

- Was the manipulation provided by a licensed chiropractor with special training in manipulation who is in good standing with the state in which he or she practices?
- Was it possible the stroke was related to some other event or pathology? In other words, is the cause and effect of manipulation clearly indicated and can manipulation be isolated as the cause?
- How recent was the manipulation in relation to the stroke?
- How many manipulations were performed in the overall study group?

Doctors have a right to ask about the safety of manipulation, and it isn't limited to the chiropractic industry. They ask the question for every type of therapeutic treatment, every drug, and every diagnostic test. Like any healthcare professional, including chiropractors, medical doctors must weigh the risk to benefit ratio for their patients.

"The Benefits Outweigh the Risks for Patients Undergoing Chiropractic Care for Neck Pain: A Prospective, Multicenter, Cohort Study." Sidney M. Rubinstein, Charlotte Leboeuf-Yde, Dirk L. Knol, Tammy E. de Koekkoek, Charles E. Pfeifle, and Maurits W. van Tulder. *Journal of Manipulative and Physiological Therapeutics.* 2007;30:408–418.

Proof Source

- The benefits of manipulation outweigh the risks for patients with neck pain.
- Side effect profile for cervical manipulation
- Efficacy of cervical manipulation for chronic recurrent cervical pain and disability

Abstract

Objective: This study describes both positive clinical outcomes and adverse events in patients treated for neck pain by a chiropractor.

Methods: This study was a prospective, multicenter, observational cohort study. Patients with neck pain of any duration who fulfilled the inclusion criteria were recruited in a practice-based study. Data were collected on the patients and from the chiropractors at baseline, the first 3 visits, and at 3 and 12 months. Clinical outcome measures included (1) neck pain in the 24 hours preceding the visit, (2) neck disability, (3) treatment satisfaction, (4) global assessment, and (5) adverse events. Recovery was defined as "completely improved" or "much better" using the global assessment scale. An adverse event was defined as either a new related complaint or a worsening of the presenting or existing complaint by >30% based upon an 11-point numerical rating scale.

Results: In all, 79 chiropractors participated, recruiting 529 subjects, representing 4,891 treatment consultations. Follow-up was possible for 90% and 92%, respectively, at 3 and 12 months. Most patients had chronic, recurrent complaints; mild to moderate disability of the neck; and a mild amount of pain at baseline; and two thirds had sought previous care for the presenting complaint in the preceding 6 months. Adverse events following any of the first 3 treatments were reported by 56%, and 13% of the study population reported these events to be severe in intensity. The most common adverse events affected the musculoskeletal system or were pain related, whereas symptoms such as tiredness, dizziness, nausea, or ringing in the ears were uncommon (<8%). Only 5 subjects (1%) reported to be much worse at 12 months. No serious adverse events were recorded during the study period. Of the patients who returned for a fourth visit, approximately half reported to be recovered, whereas approximately two thirds of the cohort were recovered at 3 and 12 months.

Conclusion: Adverse events may be common but are rarely severe in intensity. Most of the patients report recovery, particularly in the long term. Therefore, the benefits of chiropractic care for neck pain seem to outweigh the potential risks.

Promotional Strengths

- Published in *JMPT.*
- Recent publication: 2007.
- Includes 529 study subjects and 4,891 treatment visits.

- One-year prospective study assessing risk, clinical outcomes, and patient satisfaction.
- Ninety percent of patients were followed up at 3 months and 92% at 12 months with no serious adverse events reported (p. 411).
- Familiar outcome measures: Neck Disability Index (NDI), Global Assessment.
- Patients had chronic or recurrent neck pain defined as mild to moderate disability of the neck.
- Table 1 on page 411 of the study provides patient demographics:

  "Table 1 illustrates that over half of the patients had neck pain for at least 3 months and over 50% had pain greater than one year. Over 70% indicated this was at least a second occurrence and over 50% had radiating pain in the upper extremity. Patients were mostly female with an average age of 40 years old."[2]

- Table 5 on page 415 of the study provides a complete side effect profile for cervical manipulation.

  - "Adverse events reported by patients to occur 10% or higher after the 2nd visit were:

    Increased pain (29.1%)

    Increased pain >30% in the 24 hours before the visit (22%)

    Increased pain at other treatment related area (19.6%)

    Headache (10%)"[2]

  - "By the 4th visit these side effects had a dramatic decline:

    Increased pain (1.5%)

    Increased pain >30% in the 24 hours before the visit (18.6%)

    Increased pain at other related area (2.4%)

    Headache (2.8%)"[2]

  - In examining those with side effects described as intense:

    "There were none above 10%, the most frequently reported intense event was:

    - Increased pain (3.9%) after the 2nd visit which dropped to 1.5% by the 4th visit.
    - Increased pain >30% at other related area was intense for 3.1% after the second visit which dropped to 0.4% by the 4th visit.
    - Intense headaches were reported by 2.8% of the patients after the 2nd visit which dropped to 0.2% of the patients by the 4th visit.
    - In all, the only intense adverse event higher than 2% by the 4th visit was reported by 2.6% of the patients who reported an intense event of increased pain >30% in the 24 hours preceding the visit."[2]

- Table 6 on page 416 of the study illustrates the frequency of adverse events.
  - "Half of the patients reported no adverse events, and of those only 1 or 2 had events after the 2nd visit. By the 4th visit approximately ¾ of the study population had no adverse events."[2]
- Table 4 on page 414 of the study illustrates that these patients with chronic, recurrent pain with or without radiation responded positively to manipulation:

  "The total number of patients with an NDI score of moderate to severe pain declined from 187 patients to 88 patients by the 4th visit and a further decline to 70 patients at 3 months. The patients with an NDI score of none grew from 39 patients at baseline to 165 patients at 3 months."[2]

The number of patients reporting mild pain is also meaningful and certainly can be presented; however, one has to keep in mind that patients who started at baseline with an NDI of moderate or severe may account for part of the none or mild patients by the end of the study.

  "When examining the data on Global Assessment only 5 subjects in a study that had 4891 treatment consultations reported to be much worse at the end of the study, whereas, 64% of patients reported that they were much better or improved and an additional 17.3% were somewhat better."[2]

- Patient satisfaction is also available in Table 4 on page 414 of the study:

  "At the end of the visit over 80% of patients would visit a chiropractor again for their neck pain and indicated an average satisfaction score of 7.7, on a scale of 1 to 10 with 10 being the highest degree of satisfaction throughout the study. From the 4th visit to the 12 month mark patients had an average satisfaction score of approximately 33 out of 40 for their treatment with 40 being very satisfied."[2]

- A median of 8 treatments per patient was delivered (page 412 of the study) with a recovery of 48% by visit 4; 65% of patients continued to improve up to 3 months. For patients who were not recovered by 3 months, 30% went on to recover at 12 months (page 413 of the study).
- "For patients who experienced an adverse event, most reported that the discomfort was musculoskeletal in nature and 80% indicated that the adverse event did not affect their activities of daily living" (page 413 of the study).
- "In a 1-year study with 4,891 treatment visits, there were no serious neurological adverse events (page 414 of the study)."

Potential Questions and Objections

- The effectiveness does not isolate manipulation as the main factor of efficacy.
  - *"No, however, it shows that chiropractors are capable of and specialized in managing the treatment of recurrent neck pain including the use of manipulation, which demonstrated a quick response to care and without serious adverse events or the need for medication."*
- The amount of adverse reactions seems to be high.
  - *"Fifty-six percent of the patients reported either a new complaint or an increase of pain in the same general area. Of these, 75% of the complaints were musculoskeletal in nature and had no impact on patients' activities of daily living. Many of the reported adverse events were present at baseline as well, suggesting that the adverse event is part of the condition and not related to treatment. Every intervention has side effects. The side effects seen in this study were rather benign compared to adverse side effects of medications."*

    Note: If the doctor doesn't accept the comparison of the side effects of the medication to chiropractic care because they are not conducted in the same study, it is important to get the doctor's agreement that the lack of serious adverse events seen in this study of 4,891 treatment visits was indicative of the overall safety and benefits of chiropractic care, and then offer the doctor a direct comparison with the long-term study by Giles and Muller, which looked at the long-term follow-up of medication, acupuncture, and spinal manipulation mentioned in Chapter 8. If instead you chose to compare chiropractic care to physical therapy care regarding adverse events, use the same transition from this study to the Hoving RCT, which compared manual therapy, physical therapy, and continued care by a general practitioner, and which was also mentioned in Chapter 8.

Bottom Line

"This study published in JMPT with over 4,891 treatments on 591 patients illustrates the benefits of manipulation outweigh the risks for patients with mild to moderate neck pain."

"Chiropractic Manipulation and Stroke: A Population-Based Case-Control Study." Deanna M. Rothwell, Susan J. Bondy, J. Ivan Williams, and Marie-Germaine Bousser. *Stroke.* 2001;32:1054–1060.

Proof Source

- Safety of cervical manipulation relative to vertebrobasilar accidents

Abstract

Background and purpose: Several reports have linked chiropractic manipulation of the neck to dissection or occlusion of the vertebral artery. However, previous studies linking such strokes to neck manipulation consist primarily of uncontrolled case series. We designed a population-based nested case-control study to test the association.

Methods: Hospitalization records were used to identify vertebrobasilar accidents (VBAs) in Ontario, Canada, during 1993–1998. Each of 582 cases was age and sex matched to 4 controls from the Ontario population with no history of stroke at the event date. Public health insurance billing records were used to document use of chiropractic services before the event date.

Results: Results for those aged 45 years showed VBA cases to be 5 times more likely than controls to have visited a chiropractor within 1 week of the VBA (95% CI from bootstrapping, 1.32 to 43.87). Additionally, in the younger age group, cases were 5 times as likely to have had ≥3 visits with a cervical diagnosis in the month before the case's VBA date (95% CI from bootstrapping, 1.34 to 18.57). No significant associations were found for those aged ≥45 years.

Conclusions: While our analysis is consistent with a positive association in young adults, potential sources of bias are also discussed. The rarity of VBAs makes this association difficult to study despite high volumes of chiropractic treatment. Because of the popularity of spinal manipulation, high-quality research on both its risks and benefits is recommended.

Promotional Strengths

- Published in *Stroke*.
- Authors were not chiropractors, so the results are not biased.
- Large study population: *n* = 2,910 (582 had a confirmed stroke, 2,328 were matched controls).
- Research was conducted from insurance records, and this is a population-based case-control study. Michael Haneline in his book *Evidence-*

Based Chiropractic Practice[3] illustrates the following advantages and disadvantages of case-control studies:

- Advantages:

  Good for investigating rare diseases

  Can be performed quickly and inexpensively

  Useful for studying diseases with long latency period between exposure and manifestation

  Facilitate the study of multiple potential causes at once

  Existing records can often by used

- Disadvantages:

  Typically rely on patients' recall of past exposures

  Do not permit calculation of true disease rates in the population

  Difficult to validate information on exposure

  Other variables that may be associated with the disease are not controlled

- Research was supported by the Institute for Clinical Evaluative Sciences (medically oriented).

- Study reviewed all hospital records in Ontario, Canada, from 1993 to 1998 with a diagnosis of a VBA and then matched for any possible utilization of chiropractic care up to and prior to the event through public health record billings, which included universal chiropractic coverage.

- Table 1 on page 1056 of the study illustrates the timing of chiropractic services prior to the VBA and breaks up the information between two different age groups (over 45, under 45).

  - "The most important component of this table is looking at the VBA cases and the timing of their most recent cervical visit. When this is examined, only 0.5% of patients from the entire cohort had manipulation in the previous month, 0.9% had manipulation in the previous week, and only 0.7% had manipulation within the past 24 hours."

  - "When these same data are broken down by age, 3.6% under 45 years old had had a cervical visit within the past week and 1.8% had a cervical visit within the past 24 hours. For those over 45 years, 0.6% had a cervical visit within 1 month, 0.2% had a cervical visit within 1 week, and 0.4% had a cervical visit within the past 24 hours."

  - "These data suggest that manipulation is very safe for both age groups especially when compared to the risk of adverse events of medications such as nonsteroidal anti-inflammatories, a common and standard form of treatment for neck pain. As the authors point out, there is no explanation of why patients younger than 45 years old had a higher but minimal risk. Perhaps, one important and general consideration with VBAs is that patients often present initially with symptoms such as neck pain and headaches, a common complaint in a chiropractor's office."

- It is important at this point to illustrate to the doctor the following considerations doctors of chiropractic take to screen and monitor for stroke.

  - *"Chiropractors are specially trained to administer manipulation and are trained to screen for potential red flags for cerebrovascular accidents (CVAs) and to further monitor the response to treatment for warning signs. This would include but is not limited to a full health history including risk factors for stroke such as oral contraceptives, high blood pressure, smoking, and so on; a full family history including history of stroke and heart disease; detailed history of the complaint such as the location of the headache, onset, character of pain; and finally a full cervical orthopedic and neurological workup."*

    Having your examination forms and initial family and health history forms handy can help illustrate the careful workup that patients receive when visiting your chiropractic office.

  - *"In addition to this careful screening process, patients are screened for contraindications to manipulation and referred to appropriate healthcare specialists."*

  - *"During the course of treatment all patients are monitored carefully. In particular the red flag warnings of complications that are of immediate concern are referred to as the 5 Ds and 3 Ns, which include diplopia, dizziness, drop attacks, dysarthria, dysphagia; ataxia; and nausea, numbness, and nystagmus."*[4,5]

  - No significant risk for patients older than 45 years existed who would be expected to have a higher risk of CVA.

  - Unbiased study population; the study looked at every patient admitted for VBA in Ontario.

Potential Questions and Objections

- Chiropractic care is not always covered by insurance and therefore some patients represented in the study who had a stroke may not necessarily have been able to access chiropractic care. How can this study truly be controlled to determine if manipulation was associated with an increased risk of stroke?

  - *"I understand in the United States that this could certainly be true. However, this study took place in Ontario, Canada, which has a national healthcare program through which patients enjoy chiropractic benefits along with traditional medical benefits. All patients who had strokes in this study also had open access to chiropractic benefits."*

Note: In 2004, chiropractic visits were delisted from the Ontario Health Insurance Plan because of budgeting cuts, as were other ancillary services including optometry and physical therapy. Chiropractic care had been available under public funding for almost 30 years. During the study time of 1993 to 1998, patients had full access to chiropractic care through the Ontario Health Insurance Plan.

- This study reflects the fact that a risk is associated with cervical manipulation and it is difficult to tell which patients will have a stroke after manipulation. A doctor might not be able to accept this risk when patients do well with physical therapy.
    - *"The risk is minimal for all of the patients in this study especially when manipulation for back pain has proven to be more effective in treating back and neck pain compared to physical therapy."*

    Now you can move into the studies conducted on manipulation and physical therapy illustrated in Chapter 8.

    Note: Most strokes resulting from manipulation occur within 20 minutes of the treatment.[6]

Patient Types

- Patients without risk factors for CVAs and who have cervical neck pain, stiffness, headaches of any duration for which cervical manipulation would be an appropriate treatment

Bottom Line

"Manipulation as a cause of stroke is a rare event. No association could be found in stroke patients over 45 years old and for patients who are younger than 45 years, the risk of VBA associated with cervical manipulation was found to be minimal at only 5% of patients with a VBA in the month preceding their stroke."

Make sure to emphasize that the risk of stroke is not 5%, rather only 5% of patients who had a stroke or had a cervical complaint for which they sought chiropractic care in the previous month.

"An Analysis of the Etiology of Cervical Artery Dissections: 1994 to 2003." Michael T. Haneline and Gary N. Lewkovich. *Journal of Manipulative and Physiological Therapeutics.* 2005;28:617–622.

Proof Source

- Cervical manipulation and safety

Abstract

Objective: To provide a literature review of the etiologic breakdown of cervical artery dissections.

Methods: A literature search of the MEDLINE database was conducted for English-language articles published from 1994 to 2003 using the search terms *cervical artery dissection (CAD), vertebral artery dissection,* and *internal carotid artery dissection*. Articles were selected for inclusion only if they incorporated a minimum of 5 case reports of CAD and contained sufficient information to ascertain a plausible etiology.

Results: One thousand fourteen citations were identified; 20 met the selection criteria. There were 606 CAD cases reported in these studies; 321 (54%) were internal carotid artery dissection and 253 (46%) were vertebral artery dissection, not including cases with both. Three hundred seventy-one (61%) were classified as spontaneous, 178 (30%) were associated with trauma/trivial trauma, and 53 (9%) were associated with cervical spinal manipulation. If one apparently biased study is dropped from the data pool, the percentage of CADs related to cervical spinal manipulation drops to approximately 6%.

Conclusions: The case series that were reviewed in this article indicated that most CADs reported in the previous decade were spontaneous but that some were associated with trauma/trivial trauma and a minority with cervical spine manipulation. This etiologic breakdown of CAD does not differ significantly from what has been portrayed by most other authors.

Promotional Strengths

- Published in *JMPT.*
- Recent publication: 2005.
- Large study population: $n = 606$.
- Positive in that the chiropractic profession is concerned with the safety of cervical manipulation and like our medical colleagues we try to identify any correlation between cervical manipulation and stroke in an attempt to offer the safest treatment to our patients.
- Offers an etiological breakdown of VBAs based on case studies.

- Illustrates the chiropractor's in-depth knowledge of VBAs and risk factors.
- Quality figures that allow for conversation and visual correlation of the etiology of strokes. See Figures 1 (subintimal tearing), 2 (subadventitial tearing), and 3 (intramural hematoma) on page 618 of the study.
- Table I on page 619 of the study illustrates a case report review by the authors that identified the etiology of stroke:
  - *"When 606 cases of stroke over 9 years were examined, only 9% of the cases were related to manipulation, 29% were listed as being caused by a trivial action or other trauma, and the majority of which were spontaneous accounted for 61% of the cases."*[7]

    Included in these numbers is a publication that the authors noted was potentially biased against chiropractic by Norris et al. If these numbers are factored out, manipulation as a cause dropped to 6%. This is still a very low number especially when compared to spontaneous cause and trivial causes.

    This is an example of where you would want to write on your clinical copy "9%" next to the total number of 53 subjects with manipulation as an etiology (53 is 9% of 606).

- Outlines risk factors and conditions, warning signs and symptoms (pages 617–618 of the study):
  - Risk Factors

    Smoking

    Oral contraceptives

    Recent infection
  - Conditions that have a higher incidence of stroke:

    Fibromuscular dysplasia

    Marfans syndrome

    Migraine

    Hypertension

    Mild hyperhomocysteinemia
  - Warning signs and symptoms of impending dissection:

    Headache and neck pain occur in 50% to 80% of stroke patients

    Headaches are new/unusual

    Sharp

    Acute

    Tend to be unilateral on the side of dissection

    May be located in the suboccipital region

Horners syndrome

Pulsatile tinnitus in conjunction with head and/or neck pain

- Illustrates other trivial causes of stroke such as the following:

Turning the head to back up a car

Dancing

Dental work

Cervical manipulation

- Pathogenic arterial wall weakness is noted as occurring often in patients with stroke, which may put them at risk for stroke when subjected to any head or neck motion (page 620 of the study).

Potential Questions and Objections

- Chiropractic publication and authors; however, it is highly educational, which lends strong credibility to the fact that chiropractors are well educated and safe healthcare providers.

  - *"Anatomy is anatomy, etiology is etiology; chiropractors can't 'manipulate' that."*

Patient Types

- Patient with cervical neck pain or headache

Bottom Line

"Only 9% of patients who have had a stroke were found to be related to manipulation." (Again, as noted in the Rothwell study, this is not a risk of stroke in the general population; these are patients who have already had a stroke and cervical manipulation prior to the event.)

You may want to argue that if a study the authors included as part of their review was dropped, the rate fell closer to 6%. In a promotional setting it can backfire because it sounds as if you are trying to manipulate the numbers. This is not to imply that the study authors don't have good reason to support the 6% risk factor, but unless you have time to support their argument it doesn't come off right to the medical community. Nine percent is not an unacceptable number as long as you emphasize that this is not the risk of stroke for the general population; it is only representing the population that has had a stroke and an association with recent cervical manipulation.

Some neurologists have been especially critical of chiropractic care. An objection could come up that centers on a warning from a neurologist. The following study helps explain this prejudice and should be used in conjunction with one of the studies that evaluates the risk of manipulation for neck pain.

"Clinical Perceptions of the Risk of Vertebral Artery Dissection after Cervical Manipulation: The Effect of Referral Bias." Scott Haldeman, Paul Carey, Murray Townsend, and Costa Papadopoulos. *Spine.* 2002; 2:334–342.

Proof Source

- Examines provider bias by the neurology profession
- Safety of cervical manipulation

Abstract

Background context: The growing recognition of cervical manipulation as a treatment of neck pain and cervicogenic headaches has led to increased interest in potential complications that may result from this treatment approach. Recent surveys have reported that many neurologists will encounter cases of vertebral artery dissection that occur at various times after cervical manipulation, whereas most practitioners of spinal manipulation are of the opinion that these events are extremely rare. We asked the question whether these differences in perception could be explained in part by referral or selection bias.

Purpose: To assess the effect of referral bias on the differences in perceived incidence of vertebral artery dissection after cervical manipulation between neurologists and chiropractors in Canada.

Study design: This study was a retrospective review of cases where neurological symptoms consistent with cerebrovascular ischemia were reported by chiropractors in Canada.

Methods: An analysis of data from a chiropractic malpractice insurance carrier (Canadian Chiropractic Protective Association [CCPA]) and results of a survey of chiropractors was performed to determine the likelihood that a vertebral artery dissection after cervical manipulation would be reported to practicing chiropractors. This was compared with the likelihood that a neurologist would be made aware of such a complication.

Results: For the 10-year period 1988 to 1997, there were 23 cases of vertebral artery dissection after cervical manipulation reported to the CCPA that represents 85% of practicing chiropractors in Canada. Based on the survey, an estimated 134,466,765 cervical manipulations were performed during this 10-year period. This gave a calculated rate of vertebral artery dissection after manipulation of 1:5,846,381 cervical manipulations. Based on the number of practicing chiropractors and neurologists during the period of this study, 1 of every 48 chiropractors and one of every two neurologists would have been made aware of a vascular complication from cervical manipulation that was reported to the CCPA during their practice lifetime.

Conclusions: The perceived risk after cervical manipulation by chiropractors and neurologists is related to the probability that a practitioner will be made aware of such an incident. The difference in the number of chiropractors (approximately 3,840 in 1997) and neurologists (approximately 4,000 in 1997) in active practice and the fact that each patient who has a stroke after manipulation will likely be seen by only one chiropractor but by three or more neurologists partly explains the difference in experience and the perception of risk of these two professions. This selection or referral bias is important in shaping the clinical opinions of the various disciplines and distorts discussion on the true incidence of these complications of cervical manipulation. The nature of this study, however, describes the likelihood that a clinician will be made aware of such an event and cannot be interpreted as describing the actual risk of stroke after manipulation.

Promotional Strengths

- Published in *Spine*.
- Recent publication: 2002.
- Conducted by a neurologist who is also a chiropractor and therefore has intimate knowledge of etiology of stroke and the mechanism of action of manipulation.
- Ten-year study period.
- Illustrates small association of manipulation related to stroke over an extended period of time (23 patients in 10 years).

- Table 6 on page 340 of the study illustrates the breakdown of neurovascular claims.
  - *"In ten years only 23 confirmed strokes were reported to the Canadian Chiropractic Protective Association."*[8] The CCPA insures the majority of Chiropractors in Canada.
- Table 7 on page 340 of the study examines how many doctors saw the 23 patients with confirmed strokes from Table 6 of the study.
  - *"Over 219 doctors treated these 23 patients. Sixty-nine of the 219 doctors were neurologists. The authors discuss that this is not only important because of the amount of doctors seen by these patients, which overemphasizes the perception of manipulation causing stroke, but also the likelihood that at least some of these cases were presented in grand rounds as case studies."* Grand rounds are speaker presentations or case presentations conducted at medical hospitals usually during lunch hours at no charge and open to all local area physicians, they may sometimes be sponsored by a company that has an interest in the topic being discussed.
- Information is taken from medical malpractice records. This only means a claim was filed, not necessarily that the chiropractor was guilty.
- Refutes citations by neurologists who may tend to have a one-sided representation of cervical manipulation and strokes.
- Provides a nice analogy:
  - *"Chiropractors have a higher disregard for NSAIDs because they treat patients who have failed on NSAIDs. In this same manner neurologists see only the negative outcome of manipulation. The study notes no deaths from cervical manipulations but reminds providers of the estimated 3,200 deaths from NSAIDs."*[8] Note: It would *not* be well received if you told doctors that prescribing medication will kill their patients and that they should instead prescribe chiropractic manipulation. But this is useful information to illustrate to doctors that they are comfortable providing NSAIDs that have a higher rate of serious adverse events than manipulation does. It helps illustrate to doctors that manipulation is a safe choice.
- The authors on page 341 of the study note the difficulties in investigating an accurate assessment of the risk of stroke but state the following:
  - *"Because most vertebral artery dissections are spontaneous or result from traumas other than manipulation, it is not sufficient to simply assume that a stroke at some point after a manipulation is the result of manipulation."*[8]

Potential Questions and Objections

- It is difficult to find any issues when the study is conducted by a highly regarded neurologist and chiropractor. It is possible the doctor will point out that one malpractice insurance company is not reflective of an entire community.
  - The malpractice company insured 85.75% of the 4,472 licensed chiropractors in Canada in 1997.

Patient Type

- There is no patient type; rather this study is useful in overcoming an objection by a doctor who has been warned by a colleague about the dangers of stroke from manipulation.

Bottom Line

"The incidence of manipulation-related stroke has been overestimated by neurologists. This study concludes that only one chiropractor will be made aware of a specific case, whereas several neurologists will be made aware of that same case."

"Review: Inappropriate Use of the Title 'Chiropractor' and Term 'Chiropractic Manipulation' in the Peer-Reviewed Biomedical Literature." Adrian B. Wenban. *Chiropractic & Osteopathy.* 2006;14:16.

Proof Source

- Misuse of the title chiropractor in the literature

Abstract

Background: The misuse of the title "chiropractor" and term *chiropractic manipulation* in relation to injury associated with cervical spine manipulation has previously been reported in the peer-reviewed literature.

Objectives: Prospectively monitor the peer-reviewed literature for papers reporting an association between chiropractic, or chiropractic manipulation, and injury. Contact lead authors of papers that report such an association in order to determine the basis upon which the title "chiropractor" and/or term *chiropractic manipulation* was used. Document the outcome of submission of letters to the editors of journals wherein the title "chiropractor" and/or term *chiropractic manipulation* had been misused and resulted in the overreporting of chiropractic-induced injury.

Methods: One electronic database (PubMed) was monitored prospectively, via monthly PubMed searches, during a 12-month period (June 2003 to May 2004). Once relevant papers were located, they were reviewed. If the qualifications and/or profession of the care provider(s) were not apparent, an attempt was made to confirm them via direct e-mail communication with the principal researcher of each respective paper. A letter was then sent to the editor of each involved journal.

Results: A total of twenty-four different cases, spread across six separate publications, were located via the monthly PubMed searches. All twenty-four cases took place in one of two European countries. The six publications consisted of four case reports, each containing one patient; one case series, involving twenty relevant cases; and a secondary report that pertained to one of the four case reports. In each of the six publications the authors suggest the care provider was a chiropractor and that each patient received chiropractic manipulation of the cervical spine prior to developing symptoms suggestive of traumatic injury. In two of the four case reports contact with the principal researcher revealed that the care provider was not a chiropractor, as defined by the World Federation of Chiropractic. The authors of the other two case reports did not respond to my communications. In the case series, which involved twenty relevant cases, the principal researcher conceded that the term *chiropractor* had been inappropriately used and that his case series did not relate to chiropractors who had undergone appropriate formal training. The author of the secondary report, a *British Medical Journal* editor, conceded that he had misused the title "chiropractor." Letters to editors were accepted and published by all four journals to which they were sent. To date one of the four journals has published a correction.

Conclusion: The results of this year-long prospective review suggest that the words *chiropractor* and *chiropractic manipulation* are often used inappropriately by European biomedical researchers when reporting apparent associations between cervical spine manipulation and symptoms suggestive of traumatic injury. Furthermore, in those cases reported here, the spurious use of terminology seems to have passed through the peer-review process without correction. Additionally, these findings provide further preliminary evidence, beyond that already provided by Terrett, that the inappropriate use of the title "chiropractor" and term *chiropractic manipulation* may be a significant source of overreporting of the link between the care provided by chiropractors and injury. Finally, editors of peer-reviewed journals were amenable to publishing letters to editors, and to a lesser extent corrections, when authors had inappropriately used the title "chiropractor" and/or term *chiropractic manipulation*.

Promotional Strengths

- Recent publication: 2006.
- Discusses inaccurate reporting in three major categories:
  - Medical misrepresentation of the literature
  - Inaccurate reporting by medical authors
  - Inaccurate reporting by medicolegal journalists
- Illustrates bias of some medical literature, which affects not only the credibility of these studies and the associated safety but also the credibility of all future studies and systematic reviews that base their conclusions on these studies.
- Cites errors in major publications and the lack of action about the errors by the publishers.

Potential Questions and Objections

- Journal likely to be unfamiliar to doctors.
  - The word *osteopathy* is included in the journal title, which should bring legitimacy; it is clearly not a chiropractic-only text and it is available on pubmed. In addition, it should be obvious that the chiropractic profession will have to speak up for itself; the medical world isn't going to do it for us. The points the authors make can be referenced for accuracy to any doubting medical doctor.

Patient Type

- None; this is a study to utilize in response to a physician who wants to believe the negative press or allegations made in case studies that chiropractic is unsafe. In essence, you are overcoming a perceived bias about the chiropractic profession by illustrating that the bias is based on erroneous literature reporting. This article at the very least should put the *seed of doubt* in the physician's mind about the reporting on the chiropractic industry.

Bottom Line

"There is plenty of evidence that manipulation and chiropractic have been misrepresented when in fact the claims made are not always true."

Note: Be cautious when reviewing German literature. "Chiropractors" and "chiropractitioners" are not analogous. A chiropractitioner does not have formal chiropractic training. When this word is used in the literature, it can be misleading.

As mentioned earlier, one must be prepared to view a study and assess validity at all times. This is especially true when it comes to studies conducted on safety. If you find yourself presented with a study in a doctor's office that is strong and overzealous in its criticism of the safety of manipulation, remember to evaluate the following:

Who performed the manipulation?

Were the cases reviewed or was this recall by the physician?

How long until the symptoms of stroke appeared?

Was there a fair amount of supporting documentation or references?

Were both the risks and the benefits evaluated?

Was the journal peer reviewed?

Sometimes the only presenting symptoms of impending stroke are neck pain and headaches. As such, it is likely that patients will visit a chiropractor for resolution of this problem. Doctors in any specialty must listen carefully to the presenting symptoms and ask questions about onset, duration, history, family history, and so on to try to determine the cause of a patient's pain. For those with an impending stroke, it isn't always clear to any healthcare specialist. Fortunately, most patients with signs such as neck pain and headaches truly have neck pain and headaches that can be successfully treated with manipulation.

Although these patients may seek care from a chiropractor, they are just as likely to seek care from their medical doctor. It would be interesting to know how many patients who had a stroke without a history of chiropractic manipulation sought treatment for neck and headache pain from their medical doctor prior to the event. Would we fault the medical doctor for failing to diagnose impending stroke based only on these two most common and nondiscriminating symptoms? Not if the doctor provided the patient with a thorough diagnostic workup, took a thorough health and family history, and provided competent evidence-based care. This is not pointed out as a suggested promotional position to a medical doctor. It is pointed out to illustrate that because chiropractors manipulate the neck, the profession takes on the liability of such a treatment. Despite this, our malpractice rates remain some of the lowest in the healthcare industry, and despite some strong attempts by our medical foes, there is yet a credible study that has been able to suggest that the safety of cervical manipulation does not outweigh the benefit.

Safety of Lumbar Spine Manipulation

You might think this is a no-brainer, but are you aware that disc herniations were the leading cause of malpractice claims against chiropractors in 1997?[9] The relative lack of information on lumbar spine manipulation injuries in conjunction with a substantial amount of studies evaluating the efficacy of lumbar spine manipulation with large numbers of patients says it all; however, if a doctor wants a specific study looking at the safety of lumbar spine manipulation, you can use the following study.

"Safety of Spinal Manipulation in the Treatment of Lumbar Disk Herniations: A Systematic Review and Risk Assessment." Drew Oliphant. *Journal of Manipulative and Physiological Therapeutics.* 2004;27:197–210.

Proof Source

- Safety of lumbar spinal manipulation in the treatment of lumbar disc herniations (LDHs)
- Safety of manipulation compared to NSAIDs and surgery for lumbar disc herniations

Abstract

Objective: To provide a qualitative systematic review of the risk of spinal manipulation in the treatment of lumbar disk herniations (LDH) and to estimate the risk of spinal manipulation causing a severe adverse reaction in a patient presenting with LDH.

Data sources: Relevant case reports, review articles, surveys, and investigations regarding treatment of lumbar disk herniations with spinal manipulation, and adverse effects and associated risks were found with a search of the literature.

Data synthesis: Prospective/retrospective studies and review papers were graded according to quality, and results and conclusions were tabulated. From the data published, an estimate of the risk of spinal manipulation causing a clinically worsened disk herniation or cauda equina syndrome (CES) in patients presenting with LDH was calculated. This was compared with estimates of the safety of nonsteroidal anti-inflammatory drugs (NSAIDs) and surgery in the treatment of LDH.

Results: An estimate of the risk of spinal manipulation causing a clinically worsened disk herniation or CES in a patient presenting with LDH is calculated from published data to be less than 1 in 3.7 million.

Conclusion: The apparent safety of spinal manipulation, especially when compared with other accepted treatments for LDH, should stimulate its increased use in the conservative treatment plan of LDH.

Promotional Strengths

- Published in *JMPT.*
- Recent publication: 2004.
- Large study population: $n = 2,164$.
- Table 1 on page 198 of the study looks at adverse events from evidence studies conducted from 1978 through 2000.
  - *"Two thousand one hundred sixty-four patients had over 13,141 treatments. Of these lumbar patients, 117 had a LDH diagnosis. The 117 patients with a LDH had 2,010 treatments with no major or permanent adverse reactions."*
- Table 3 on page 200 of the study lists four previously published papers and the estimated risk of cauda equina syndrome and LDH resulting from spinal manipulation.

- ■ *"The papers with the highest quality score also had similar risk evaluations for cauda equina syndrome of 1 in 100 or 128 million manipulations."*
- Table 8 on page 204 of the study provides the population risk of cauda equina syndrome.
  - ■ *"The risk of cauda equina syndrome resulting from lumbar spinal manipulation is less than 1 in 3.7 million."*
- Discusses and briefly highlights literature that explains a possible mechanism of action of disc ruptures relative to spinal manipulation (pages 206 to 207 of the study). There are no pictures to help with a verbal presentation; however, this can be overcome with the use of a spine model for the doctor who asks for the etiology of LDHs.
- Contains analogies to other common treatments and puts the risk of adverse events of manipulation in perspective to other commonly accepted treatments such as NSAIDs and surgery (pages 205 and 206 of the study).
  - ■ Spinal manipulation is at least 37,000 to 148,000 times safer than NSAIDs and 55,500 to 444,000 times safer than surgery for LDH.[10]
  - ■ Cauda equina syndrome is at least 7,400 to 37,000 times more likely to occur as a complication of surgery than of spinal manipulation.[10]

Potential Questions and Objections

- This is a thesis paper.
  - ■ *"This paper was prepared as part of a master's thesis and is copyrighted by a chiropractic college and was accepted for publication in a reputable and peer-reviewed journal. In addition, Dr. Oliphant is a fellow of the College of Chiropractic Orthopedists (Canada), which means that he has participated in additional education and has passed a separate board examination to attain such status."*
- How did the author arrive at the numbers for safety compared to the safety of NSAIDs and surgery? (It is recommended that you write the following equations in your copy of the study.)
  - ■ "Regarding NSAIDs, the safety of manipulation is 1 in 3.7 million patients who could be expected to have an adverse event. By taking the 3.7 million associated with manipulation (1 in 3.7 million risk of LDH) and multiplying it by 1% and 4% of significant complications that occurs with NSAID users, you get:

$$1 \times 3.7 \times 10,000 = 37,000, \text{ and}$$
$$4 \times 3.7 \times 10,000 = 148,000.$$

"Regarding surgery, these calculations are repeated for the surgical group using 1.5% and 12% significant risk of surgery to reveal that

$$1.5 \times 3.7 \times 10{,}000 = 55{,}500, \text{ and}$$
$$12 \times 3.7 \times 10{,}000 = 444{,}000.$$

"For cauda equina and surgery, 0.2% to 1% of surgeries can result in cauda equina. We can use the following equations to find the results:

$$0.2 \times 3.7 \times 10{,}000 = 7{,}400, \text{ and}$$
$$1 \times 3.7 \times 10{,}000 = 37{,}000."$$

Patient Types

- Patients with LDH
- Patients with lumbar pain and stiffness

Bottom Line

"Manipulation has a lower risk compared to other accepted treatment protocols for lumbar disc herniation and is a safe and effective treatment for lower back pain."

Note: The large study conducted by Dr. Haas on Lower Back Pain covered in Chapter 8 that included patients with leg pain would also be a proof source on safety of manipulation for the lower back.

Doctors should be educated that you are aware of the warning signs of a worsening of a disc herniation and cauda equina. Explain to the doctor that you are aware of the warning signs and monitor every patient for the following:

Bowel and bladder dysfunction, especially urinary retention

Saddle anesthesia

Bilateral leg weakness

Sensory changes

A Note on Informed Consent

Another issue that might arise that falls under safety is the perception that because our patients sign informed consent forms we are asking them to absolve us of all liability should something happen. This is not accurate. A doctor should understand that informed consent means that we have discussed the diagnosis, treatment options, and associated complications in a conversational dialogue for each condition that the patient has and that the patient has

Table 9-1 *Malpractice Claims by Healthcare Specialty*

Profession	Claims between 9/1990 and 8/13/2007	Average claims per year by profession (rough estimate)
Chiropractor	4,982	293
Doctor of osteopathy	14,301	841
Dentist	39,389	2,317
Physician (MD)	226,684	13,334

Source: Adapted from the National Practitioner Data Bank (NPDB). US Department of Health and Human Services. Available at http://www.npdb-hipdb.hrsa.gov.

given his or her consent to undergo treatment and is aware of the associated risks. Informed consent is required for any of a multitude of minor procedures that patients undergo in thousands of medical offices around the country.

Malpractice

When considering the safety of manipulation, who knows better than malpractice companies? Chiropractors have one of the lowest malpractice premiums. According to Brady in 1994[11] and the Medical Liability Monitor in 1994[12], the percentages of malpractice suits for chiropractors are significantly lower than the percentages of the medical and legal fields. Malpractice suits, as doctors also know, do not mean guilt or negligence, but they are a reflection of the seriousness and complications that arise from provider care. Chiropractors not only enjoy low premiums but also a low number of malpractice claims. Take, for instance, the information in Table 9–1, which is adapted from the National Practitioner Data Bank.

Remember, when a study is evaluated for the safety of manipulation, be it promotional or best practices, cervical or lumbar, one must consider two critical components:

1. Did the authors provide support that the manipulation that was provided had a distinct and causal relationship to the stroke?
2. Was the manipulation provided by a qualified and licensed healthcare professional with specialized training in manipulative technique?

The safety of manipulation and the etiology of the more serious adverse events resulting from manipulation are extremely complicated subjects. Therefore, when presenting the data, let the numbers speak for themselves. There is no need for salesmanship here. Adverse events relative to manipulation and medication and surgery are a far safer bet for credibility.

REFERENCES

1. Chiropractic Report. May 2001. Safety and Effectiveness of Cervical Manipulation: Addressing the Gap Between Perception and Reality. May 2001. Vol. 15. No. 3. David Chapman-Smith.

2. Rubinstein S, Leboeuf-Yde C, Knol D, de Koekkoek T, Pfeifle C, van Tulder M. The benefits outweigh the risks for patients undergoing chiropractic care for neck pain: a prospective, multicenter, cohort study. *J Manipulative Physiol Ther.* 2007;30:408–418.

3. Haneline M. *Evidence-Based Chiropractic Practice.* 2007. Sudbury, MA: Jones and Bartlett.

4. Terrett AGJ. *Current Concepts: Vertebrobasilar Complications Following Spinal Manipulation.* West Des Moines, IA: NCMIC Group, Inc.; 2001.

5. Haneline MT, Lewkovich G. Chiropractic manipulation and cervical artery dissection. *JACA.* January 2007:20–26.

6. Haldeman et al. Research letter: arterial dissections following cervical manipulation: the chiropractic experience. *CMAJ.* 2001;165(7):905–906.

7. Haneline M, Lewkovich G. An analysis of the etiology of cervical artery dissections: 1994 to 2003. *J Manipulative Physiol Ther.* 2005;28:617–622.

8. Haldeman S, Carey P, Townsend M, Papadopoulos C. Clinical perceptions of the risk of vertebral artery dissection after cervical manipulation: the effect of referral bias. *Spine.* 2002;2:334–342.

9. Jagbandhansingh MP. Most common causes of chiropractic malpractice lawsuits. *J Manipulative Physiol Ther.* 1997;20:60–64.

10. Oliphant D. Safety of spinal manipulation in the treatment of lumbar disk herniations: a systematic review and risk assessment. *J Manipulative Physiol Ther.* 2004;27:197–210.

11. Brady T. Defensive and offensive approaches to chiropractic lawsuits. *J Amer Chiropr Assoc.* 1994;32(11)39–47. Quoted from MGI of America: The Chiropractic Profession and Its Research and Education Programs. Available at www.fsu.edu/~chiro/1554-8.pdf. p. 4-15.

12. Medical Liability Monitor. Defensive and offensive approaches to chiropractic lawsuits. *J Amer Chiropr Assoc.* 1994;32(11)39–47. Quoted from MGI of America: The Chiropractic Profession and Its Research and Education Programs. Available at www.fsu.edu/~chiro/1554-8.pdf. p. 4–15.

Chapter 10

Cost-Effectiveness of Chiropractic Care

I n recent years, research has provided the chiropractic profession with an arsenal of cost-effectiveness studies for the chiropractic management of neuromuscular disorders to present to medical doctors. Several are also applicable in a managed care or political promotional setting.

The rising cost of managed care has resulted in increased costs for employers and subsequently for employees, with higher premiums, copays, and deductibles. Providers of care have seen their reimbursements dwindle and are forced to spend more time doing administrative tasks. Doctors are forced to see more patients in less time.

Consumers are demanding alternative health care, and despite the increase in out-of-pocket expenses chiropractic has continued to grow.[1] Managed care is attempting to control costs and meet consumer demand, so the bottom line as it pertains to chiropractic is whether or not having chiropractic coverage is as effective as managing pain compared to allopathic care and, in doing so, is it safe and cost-effective?

Research has demonstrated that manipulation is effective at treating certain neuromuscular-skeletal (NMS) conditions; however, according to some research, it has yet to be proven that it is better at doing so than medical care is in the long term. As such, safety and cost-effectiveness studies become major players in the battle for market share and in deciding the role chiropractors will play in the future of health care. Many past philosophies of chiropractic professionals encouraged "maintenance" care for all patients, which did not help the chiropractic profession today and in fact jeopardizes our current professional standing in health care. The studies that are included in this chapter look at many of these aspects and specifically question whether chiropractic care will decrease or increase healthcare costs.

It is critically important to understand that the efficacy data included in this text look at manipulation, a treatment tool that is finding its way into the treatment arsenal of a growing array of providers. Cost-effectiveness data look primarily at the chiropractic profession. It cannot be underestimated in the importance of how chiropractors as a profession manage patient care. It is clear that many of our patients request maintenance treatments. What is not clear is the evidence that supports maintenance treatment and the expectation by chiropractic providers and patients that insurance should bear the financial burden of elective care. The lack of evidence supporting this philosophy undermines the importance chiropractors could play in the healthcare arena.

This chapter is useful in illustrating cost concerns or objections that physicians may have when referring their patients for chiropractic care. It is also useful for any managed care reimbursement issues that come up in your office and any political efforts that you seek with local and state legislators in your community. Baby boomers are especially focused on the costs of chiropractic care. There is a tremendous amount of information available on the cost-effectiveness of chiropractic care. As stated in other chapters, the reports selected for this text are routinely available in Pub Med and the Manual Alternative and Natural Therapy Index System or through government agencies and are reasonably recent in their publication dates. When thinking of patient types, keep the following in mind:

- These studies will most likely be an extension of another study to validate the cost. As such, you should carry the patient type through to these data.
- These studies may also be brought out on their own where the doctor has a cost concern or objection. Again, the original patient type should be used.

"Comparative Analysis of Individuals with and Without Chiropractic Coverage: Patient Characteristics, Utilization, and Costs." A. P. Legorreta, R. D. Metz, C. F. Nelson, S. Ray, H. O. Chernicoff, and N. A. Dinubile. *Archives of Internal Medicine.* 2004;164:1985–1992.

Proof Source

- Cost-effectiveness
- Decreased utilization of X-rays and magnetic resonance imaging (MRI) compared to medical providers
- Safety and patient satisfaction

Abstract

Background: Back pain accounts for more than $100 billion in annual U.S. healthcare costs and is the second leading cause of physician visits and hospitalizations. This study ascertains the effect of systematic access to chiropractic care on the overall and neuromusculoskeletal-specific consumption of healthcare resources within a large managed care system.

Methods: A 4-year retrospective claims data analysis comparing more than 700,000 health plan members with an additional chiropractic coverage benefit and 1 million members of the same health plan without the chiropractic benefit.

Results: Members with chiropractic insurance coverage, compared with those without coverage, had lower annual total healthcare expenditures ($1,463 vs $1,671 per member per year, $P < 0.001$). Having chiropractic coverage was associated with a 1.6% decrease ($P = 0.001$) in total annual healthcare costs at the health plan level. Back pain patients with chiropractic coverage, compared with those without coverage, had lower utilization (per 1,000 episodes) of plain radiographs (17.5 vs 22.7, $P < 0.001$), low back surgery (3.3 vs 4.8, $P < 0.001$), hospitalizations (9.3 vs 15.6, $P < 0.001$), and magnetic resonance imaging (43.2 vs 68.9, $P < 0.001$). Patients with chiropractic coverage, compared with those without coverage, also had lower average back pain episode-related costs ($289 vs $399, $P < 0.001$).

Conclusions: Access to managed chiropractic care may reduce overall healthcare expenditures through several effects, including (1) positive risk selection; (2) substitution of chiropractic for traditional medical care, particularly for spine conditions; (3) more conservative, less invasive treatment profiles; and (4) lower health service costs associated with managed chiropractic care. Systematic access to managed chiropractic care not only may prove to be clinically beneficial but also may reduce overall healthcare costs.

Promotional Strengths

- Published in the *Archives of Internal Medicine.*
- Recent publication: 2004.
- Authors are MD/DC, some of whom work with a large managed care organization.
- Large study population: $n = 1.7$ M.
- Long-term study: 4 years.
- Participant, nonparticipant retrospective longitudinal study design. In simple terms: A managed care company had total access to its own records to compare a large population of patients with and without chiropractic benefits and the effect the benefits had on the insurance companies' bottom-line finances. From a business perspective, who better to evaluate the cost-effectiveness of chiropractic care for one of the most expensive healthcare conditions in the United States than those who are actually making the payments in a for-profit company.

- Safety, efficacy, and patient satisfaction are confirmed on the first page of the study, again by a managed care company that has a strong financial interest.
- Physical therapy (PT) and prescription medications were not included in the comparator costs, and the findings are still significant in favor of chiropractic.
- Figure 1 on page 1989 of the study examines the annual total cost reduction between the chiropractic group and nonchiropractic group.
  - *"Adding chiropractic benefits did not increase NMS healthcare expenditure. In fact, it decreased it by $208 per member/per year. This was statistically significant."*
- Figure 2 on page 1989 of the study examines the overall medical expenditures between the two groups including hospital costs:
  - *"The amount of per member per year expenditure for chiropractic coverage was only 1% of the total cost per year. The total medical costs when compared between those with and without chiropractic benefits were lower by $361.00 or 13%, a statistically significant difference in favor of chiropractic care." (Authors also discuss this on page 1988.)*
- Figure 3 on page 1990 of the study examines the episode of care utilization both from a cost per episode and cost per patient:
  - *"When the cost per episode and the cost per patient data were examined for a 4-year period, members with chiropractic coverage for NMS conditions had statistically significant lower costs."*
- Figure 4 on page 1990 of the study examines the cost of X-rays, MRI, low back surgery, and inpatient stays between the chiropractic and nonchiropractic groups:
  - *"Neuromuscular patients with chiropractic coverage had statistically significant lower utilization of X-rays and MRIs and a statistically significant lower need for lumbar surgery and inpatient stays."*
- Figure 5 on page 1990 of the study examines medical care substitution when patients have access to chiropractic care:
  - *"This graph represents the choice patients make between chiropractic and medical providers for neuromuscular disorders that is dependent on their insurance benefits. Patients without chiropractic benefits sought medical care from MDs; however, a statistically significant shift was observed when patients had chiropractic access with a decrease in medical physician care for the neck and back. This suggests a substitution of DC care for MD care."* (It is noted that during the same period a very high rate was observed for patients seeking chiropractic care from network providers for back and neck conditions.)

- The authors make an interesting point that can be utilized with employers who desire a healthier workforce. In the comments section on page 1991 of the study, the authors point out that offering chiropractic benefits may attract younger and healthier individuals, and that employees who maintain healthier lifestyles may seek out employers who offer access to complementary care companies.
- Another important point is made by the authors on page 1991 of the study: *"In our study population of 0.7 million members who had chiropractic coverage in the medical plan, we estimated an annual reduction of approximately $16 million as a result of lower utilization high-cost items. . . . The estimated cost saving appears to more than offset the amount spent to cover the associated costs of the chiropractic benefit."*[2]

Potential Questions and Objections

- X-rays and MRIs had higher utilization for patients without chiropractic coverage because the patients' conditions with chiropractic coverage were not as severe and the patients did not have as many comorbid conditions.
  - *"Yes; however, the authors did address this and only 2% in the difference of severity between the two groups was noted and was not statistically significant"* (page 1991 of the study). The option to move into an efficacy study or remind the doctor of a previous conversation about an efficacy study for a moderate to severe patient is also an option that can overcome this objection. In studies comparing chiropractic and medical management of patients, all studies note the lower utilization of X-rays and MRIs by chiropractors without compromising safety. This is perhaps because chiropractors are comfortable treating these conditions.

Patient Types

- Patients with managed care coverage and neuromuscular conditions
- Patients without any healthcare coverage to decrease their direct and indirect out-of-pocket expenses

Bottom Line

"Patients with chiropractic access have lower medical costs associated with the treatment of NMS conditions, which means that the savings of chiropractic care more than covers the cost of providing chiropractic care."

"Cost-Effectiveness of Medical and Chiropractic Care for Acute and Chronic Low Back Pain." Mitchell Haas, Rajiv Sharma, and Miron Stano. *Journal of Manipulative and Physiological Therapeutics.* 2005;28:555–563.

Proof Source

- Cost-effectiveness of chiropractic care compared to medical care for acute and chronic lower back
- Patient satisfaction

Abstract

Objectives: To identify relative provider costs, clinical outcomes, and patient satisfaction for the treatment of low back pain (LBP).

Methods: This was a practice-based, nonrandomized, comparative study of patients self-referring to 60 doctors of chiropractic and 111 medical doctors in 51 chiropractic and 14 general practice community clinics over a 2-year period. Patients were included if they were at least 18 years old, ambulatory, and had low back pain of mechanical origin ($n = 2,780$). Outcomes were (standardized) office costs, office costs plus referral costs for office-based care and advanced imaging, pain, functional disability, patient satisfaction, physical health, and mental health evaluated at 3 and 12 months after the start of care. Multiple regression analysis was used to correct for baseline differences between provider types.

Results: Chiropractic office costs were higher for both acute and chronic patients ($P < 0.01$). When referrals were included, there were no significant differences in either group between provider types ($P > 0.20$). Acute and chronic chiropractic patients experienced better outcomes in pain, functional disability, and patient satisfaction ($P < 0.01$); clinically important differences in pain and disability improvement were found for chronic patients only.

Conclusions: Chiropractic care appeared relatively cost-effective for the treatment of chronic LBP. Chiropractic and medical care performed comparably for acute patients. Practice-based clinical outcomes were consistent with systematic reviews of spinal manipulation efficacy: Manipulation-based therapy is at least as good as and, in some cases, better than other therapeusis. This evidence can guide physicians, payers, and policymakers in evaluating chiropractic as a treatment option for low back pain.

Promotional Strengths

- Published in *JMPT.*
- Recent publication date: 2005.
- Large study population: $n = 2,780$.
- Part of a large prospective longitudinal study discussed in the previous chapter on efficacy.
- Funded by the Health Resources and Services Administration, Department of Health and Human Resources.
- Table 1 on page 558 of the study illustrates the patient demographics, some of which were presented previously for the efficacy portion of this paper. In this study, patients without insurance or those who paid on their own were most prevalent in the chiropractic groups.
- Table 2 on page 559 of the study illustrates total costs, pain and disability scores, as well as patient satisfaction with care.
  - *"When the mean costs of care were compared to the total cost and the office costs, one trend was clear. Chiropractic office costs compared to total costs had only a $6 to $12 difference in the acute and chronic groups during the 3- and 12-month time period. However, MD office costs compared to total costs for the same time period had much greater differences that ranged from $51 to $135 for each of the groups. These values indicate referral and advanced imaging accounted for a large fraction of the mean total costs for MD-treated acute and chronic patients."*

    Note: It helps to illustrate these differences by writing the values down on your copy of the study. For instance, in the 3-month data for chronic patients, the difference in office costs from total costs was $6.00 ($180 of total costs minus $174 for office costs = $6 difference). Providing these differences in each treatment group for both the 3- and 12-month data provides the ranges used to explain this table.
- Table 3 on page 559 of the study illustrates the adjusted mean differences in costs and outcomes between the MD and DC groups.
  - *"A positive value indicates a greater cost or better outcome for chiropractic patients. For chronic patients, the value of chiropractic care is notable. The total additional cost of $5 provided statistically significant improvements in pain and disability at the 3-month mark and only $1 for a statistically significant advantage in pain and disability at the 12-month mark for chiropractic patients. Patient satisfaction was higher for chiropractic patients."*

- Clarify that the numbers included for chiropractic care included physical therapy modalities, but that physical therapy referrals were not included by medical doctors (discussed on page 560 of the study).
  - *"Chiropractors will administer treatments appropriate for the condition, which could include physical modalities. These cost data include physiotherapy for the chiropractic group, but not for physiotherapy costs that are accrued when the doctor refers the patients out for physiotherapy care. Despite this the findings still showed (Table 2 on page 559 of the study) that the total mean cost for chronic patients in the chiropractic group was $180 versus $212 for the chronic patients in the medical group. This is important when one considers that chronic back pain treatments are responsible for much of the healthcare spending compared to acute lower back pain."*

Potential Questions and Objections

- The cost data illustrate that there is an advantage for chronic patients but not acute patients who paid $161 for a DC office visit and only $90 for an MD visit.
  - *"This is true; however, taking into account the total office costs, patients in the DC group had only a $30 difference at the 3-month mark. This illustrates that office costs alone do not present the entire picture. To further explain it is important to note that these medical costs for office visits do not include physical therapy, but chiropractors routinely perform physical therapy, which is included in the DC office costs. As the authors point out, advanced imaging and physical therapy costs associated with lower back disorders appear to equal out the cost differences between the medical and chiropractic costs. In addition, pharmacological management is also not included and would greatly affect the MD care costs, especially if you take into account the greater frequency of adverse events such as GI bleeding that occurs with medication and the medical management costs associated with treating these side effects."*

Patient Types

- Patients with a limit or annual cap on their chiropractic or PT benefits
- Patients who might pay cash

Bottom Line

"Chiropractic care is cost-effective for the treatment of acute and chronic lower back pain with greater overall patient satisfaction and lower number of office visits to achieve efficacy."

"United Kingdom Back pain Exercise And Manipulation (UK BEAM) Randomised Trial: Cost Effectiveness of Physical Treatments for Back Pain in Primary Care." UK BEAM Trial Team. *British Medical Journal.* 2004;329:1377.

Proof Source

- Cost-effectiveness

Abstract

Objective: To assess the cost effectiveness of adding spinal manipulation, exercise classes, or manipulation followed by exercise ("combined treatment") to "best care" in general practice for patients consulting with low back pain.

Design: Stochastic cost utility analysis alongside pragmatic randomised trial with factorial design.

Setting: 181 general practices and 63 community settings for physical treatments around 14 centres across the United Kingdom.

Participants: 1,287 (96%) of 1,334 trial participants.

Main outcome measures: Healthcare costs, quality adjusted life years (QALYs), and cost per QALY over 12 months.

Results: Over one year, mean treatment costs relative to "best care" were £195 ($360; €279; 95% credibility interval £85 to £308) for manipulation, £140 (£3 to £278) for exercise, and £125 (£21 to £228) for combined treatment. All three active treatments increased participants' average QALYs compared with best care alone. Each extra QALY that combined treatment yielded relative to best care cost £3800; in economic terms it had an "incremental cost-effectiveness ratio" of £3800. Manipulation alone had a ratio of £8700 relative to combined treatment. If the NHS was prepared to pay at least £10,000 for each extra QALY (lower than previous recommendations in the United Kingdom), manipulation alone would probably be the best strategy. If manipulation was not available, exercise would have an incremental cost-effectiveness ratio of £8300 relative to best care.

Conclusions: Spinal manipulation is a cost effective addition to "best care" for back pain in general practice. Manipulation alone probably gives better value for money than manipulation followed by exercise.

Promotional Strengths

- Published in the *British Medical Journal.*
- Recent publication: 2004.
- Mixed group of authors including MDs.
- Large study population: $n = 1,287$.
- Long-term cost analysis: 1 year.
- Table 1 on page 2 of the study illustrates the difference in the cost of a unit of healthcare by different provider types.
  - *"Chiropractic care (initial consultation and follow-up treatments) were similar to other provider office visits. For instance, a 20-minute follow-up chiropractic treatment session had an associated cost of £12.17, which is slightly less than a physiotherapy visit at £15.00 and a general practitioner (GP) visit at £21.50."*
- Table 3 on page 3 of the study illustrates the QALY.
  - *"The QALY is used to quantify the benefit of an intervention by measuring both the quality and quantity of life lived. In addition, a scoring process was utilized to value the quality of life with a patient-completed questionnaire referred to as the EQ-5D. The EQ-5D is a scale that examines mobility, self-care, usual activities, pain–discomfort, and anxiety–depression and is scored as 0 = death and 1 = perfect health. A higher number denotes a greater improvement. Manipulation alone had the highest mark of 0.041."*
- Table 4 on page 4 of the study provides a visual graph that nicely illustrates the cost-effectiveness ratio between each of the treatment groups. The probability that manipulation alone is best is illustrated in the middle panel.

Potential Questions and Objections

- Physical therapists were not allowed to administer palliative care such as electrical muscle stimulation and ultrasound heat. The findings may have been different if they were able to use these therapies.
  - *"Neither were chiropractors who are also trained to deliver such palliative treatments."*

Patient Types

- Patients whose insurance may have a cap on limits or benefits
- Patients who may have to pay out of pocket
- Managed care reimbursements

Bottom Line

"In addition to assessing efficacy, the UK BEAM Trial Team looked at the associated costs relative to the benefits. The authors concluded that manipulation alone probably gives better value for the money than does manipulation followed by exercise."

"Utilization, Cost, and Effects of Chiropractic Care on Medicare Program Costs." July 2001. Executive Summary. Available from the ACA. Available at www.ACATODAY.com

---

Proof Source

- Cost of care for baby boomers

Abstract

This study examines the utilization, cost, and effects of chiropractic services on Medicare program costs. In the course of this investigation, service utilization and program payments for Medicare beneficiaries who were treated by doctors of chiropractic are compared with similar data for beneficiaries treated by other provider types. The results strongly suggest that chiropractic care significantly reduces per beneficiary costs to the Medicare program. The results also suggest that chiropractic services could play a role in reducing costs of Medicare reform and/or a new prescription drug benefit.

Promotional Strengths

- Government study.
- Large study population: $n = 5.8$ million (1.5 million treated with chiropractic and 4.3 million treated without chiropractic care).
- On page 5 of the report, builds upon research conducted by the Department of Defense that illustrated that chiropractic services had
  - Better health outcomes
  - Higher satisfaction
  - Lower costs

- The Department of Defense study included a section on the elderly; this report builds upon this section and targets cost-effectiveness for baby boomers.
- Table 2 on page 8 of the report provides a summary of costs associated with the beneficiary seeing or not seeing a chiropractor:
  - *"Those who did see a chiropractor had 37% lower average payment per claim and close to a 50% reduction in average payment per beneficiary."*
- Table 3 on page 9 of the report extracts data from Table 2 and looks at all musculoskeletal-related claims:
- *"Those who did see a chiropractor had almost a 70% reduction in average payment per claim and approximately 40% reduction in average payments per beneficiary."*
- Table 5 on page 12 of the report is a nice visual aid that illustrates the amount per encounter. Encounter does not mean a visit, rather it is defined as follows: "A chronologically contiguous episode of care at a particular provider type from a single Standard Analytical Public Use File (SAF). Because date of service is not listed on the claims, the chronological order was determined by using incurred quarter and claim receipt date."[3]
  - *"The table depicts that for the first encounter provided for a beneficiary seen by a doctor of chiropractic the Medicare payment per beneficiary is slightly higher by $34.40. However, when the second and third encounters are examined, the beneficiaries treated by a chiropractor had fewer encounters and fewer costs."*
- Table 9 on page 17 of the report represents the most stringent look at the Medicare population in that it includes all patients with neuromuscular claims but excludes patients in skilled nursing and hospice care:
  - *"Beneficiaries seen by a chiropractor enjoyed a 60% reduction in average payment per claim."*
- The conclusions reached by the authors are stated on page 17 of the report: "In conclusion, these results strongly suggest that Chiropractic care reduces per beneficiary costs to the Medicare program under current law."[3]

Potential Questions and Objections

- There are no true efficacy data, only implied efficacy, that this is a worthwhile benefit.
  - *"This is a continuation of a Department of Defense study in which it was determined that users had better health outcomes and which allowed for the integration of chiropractic into the Department of*

Defense. Geriatric patients were included as part of that study. In addition, beneficiaries who had access to chiropractic care had lower durable medical costs, home health costs, outpatient costs, and professional costs, which implies efficacy."

Patient Types

- Baby boomers with neuromuscular complaints
- Patients concerned with out-of-pocket costs
- Medicare patients

Bottom Line

"Chiropractic care significantly lowers costs for a population with fixed incomes and concerned with healthcare costs."

"Clinical Utilization and Cost Outcomes from an Integrative Medicine Independent Physician Association: An Additional 3-Year Update." Richard L. Sarnat, James Winterstein, and Jerrilyn A. Cambron. *Journal of Manipulative and Physiological Therapeutics.* 2007;30:263–269.

Proof Source

- Chiropractors performance and impact on hospital admissions, pharmaceuticals, and surgical rates when acting as primary care physicians. (With the expected shortage of physicians in the next few years, the doors may be opening for chiropractors to be accepted as primary care physicians.)
- For presenting to managed care organizations and politicians

Abstract

Objective: Our initial report analyzed clinical and cost utilization data from the years 1999 to 2002 for an integrative medicine independent physician association (IPA) whose primary care physicians (PCPs) were exclusively doctors of chiropractic. This report updates the subsequent utilization data from the IPA for the years 2003 to 2005 and includes first time comparisons in data points among PCPs of different licensures who were oriented toward complementary and alternative medicine (CAM).

Methods: Independent physician association–incurred claims and stratified random patient surveys were descriptively analyzed for clinical utilization, cost offsets, and member satisfaction compared with conventional medical IPA normative values. Comparisons to our original publication's comparative blinded data, using nonrandom matched comparison groups, were descriptively analyzed for differences in age/sex demographics and disease profiles to examine sample bias.

Results: Clinical and cost utilization based on 70,274 member-months over a 7-year period demonstrated decreases of 60.2% in-hospital admissions, 59.0% hospital days, 62.0% outpatient surgeries and procedures, and 85% pharmaceutical costs when compared with conventional medicine IPA performance for the same health maintenance organization product in the same geography and time frame.

Conclusion: During the past 7 years, and with a larger population than originally reported, the CAM-oriented PCPs using a nonsurgical/nonpharmaceutical approach demonstrated reductions in both clinical and cost utilization when compared with PCPs using conventional medicine alone. Decreased utilization was uniformly achieved by all CAM-oriented PCPs, regardless of their licensure. The validity and generalizability of this observation are guarded given the lack of randomization, lack of statistical analysis possible, and potentially biased data in this population.

Promotional Strengths

- Published in *JMPT*.
- Recent publication: 2007.
- Authors were MD/DC.
- Long-term follow-up: 7 years.
- Large study population: $n = 70,274$ member months.
- Supports the role of CAM providers as primary care providers, which in conjunction with the forecasted shortage of medical doctors may be a key promotional feature.
- The study consisted of two matched control groups, which means that there was less potential for sample bias.
- Table 2 on page 266 of the study illustrates well-patient diagnostic coding between the two groups:
  - *"Alternative Medicine Integration's (AMI's) providers illustrated an increased percentage of active disease coding compared to conventional medical IPA groups listed as comparison groups I and II. This*

means that the nontraditional approach was successful in treating patients who might otherwise be considered to be overly worried or perhaps hypochondriacal."

- Table 3 on page 266 of the study illustrates that CAM provided from 1999 to 2005 resulted in
  - *"60% less hospital admissions, 62% fewer surgeries, and 85% less pharmaceutical usage."*
- Table 4 on page 267 of the study illustrates that cost savings were more than expected.
  - *"The column of percentage units saved is impressive for each year and illustrates that utilization fell below the predicted value in all 7 years."*
- Patient satisfaction is discussed under the Quality of Care heading on page 267 of the study. The AMI group participants received higher marks compared to the health maintenance organization groups.
- Page 268 of the study illustrates under practical applications that chiropractic PCPs managed 60% of their patients without requiring a referral to a conventional medical specialist.

Potential Questions and Objections

- This study was not necessarily chiropractic specific because osteopaths were also included from 2002. It is also not back pain specific.
  - *"This study examines a different approach to care by managing patients from a holistic approach rather than a traditional approach for common complaints within a particular scope of practice. The end result was reduced medical costs and higher patient satisfaction."*
- This is not a study that can be applied to every setting.
  - "Yes, further trials are needed. It is, however, a very good business model of success in controlling costs for this particular group."

Patient Types

- This study does not have an associated patient type, but rather is a good study to illustrate to hospitals and managed care organizations.

Bottom Line

"Chiropractors are qualified to be primary care physicians, which in this study lowered healthcare costs for hospital admissions and stays, surgery, and pharmaceuticals compared to the conventional medicine control group and provided greater patient satisfaction."

"Cost-Effectiveness of Physiotherapy, Manual Therapy, and General Practitioner Care for Neck Pain: Economic Evaluation Alongside a Randomised Controlled Trial." Ingeborg B. C. Korthals-de Bos, Jan L. Hoving, Maurits W. van Tulder, et al. *British Medical Journal.* 2003;326:1–6.

Proof Source

- Indirect and direct costs of manual therapy for the cervical spine
- Head-to-head cost data comparing DC, PT, and GP care
- Safety

Abstract

Objective: To evaluate the cost effectiveness of physiotherapy, manual therapy, and care by a general practitioner for patients with neck pain.

Design: Economic evaluation alongside a randomised controlled trial.

Setting: Primary care.

Participants: 183 patients with neck pain for at least two weeks recruited by 42 general practitioners and randomly allocated to manual therapy ($n = 60$, spinal mobilization), physiotherapy ($n = 59$, mainly exercise), or general practitioner care ($n = 64$, counseling, education, and drugs).

Main outcome measures: Clinical outcomes were perceived recovery, intensity of pain, functional disability, and quality of life. Direct and indirect costs were measured by means of cost diaries that were kept by patients for one year. Differences in mean costs between groups, cost effectiveness, and cost utility ratios were evaluated by applying non-parametric bootstrapping techniques.

Results: The manual therapy group showed a faster improvement than the physiotherapy group and the general practitioner care group up to 26 weeks, but differences were negligible by follow-up at 52 weeks. The total costs of manual therapy (€447; £273; $402) were around one third of the costs of physiotherapy (€1297) and general practitioner care (€1379). These differences were significant: $P < 0.01$ for manual therapy versus physiotherapy and manual therapy versus general practitioner care and $P = 0.55$ for general practitioner care versus physiotherapy. The cost effectiveness ratios and the cost utility ratios showed that manual therapy was less costly and more effective than physiotherapy or general practitioner care.

Conclusions: Manual therapy (spinal mobilisation) is more effective and less costly for treating neck pain than physiotherapy or care by a general practitioner.

Promotional Strengths

- Published in the *British Medical Journal.*
- Recent publication: 2003.
- Authors: MD.
- Good study population: $n = 183$.
- Cost-efficacy data administered alongside a clinical trial for neck pain.
- Compares manual therapy cost to physiotherapy and medical care.
- Long term (patients completed a cost diary of 52 weeks).
- Although it is not U.S.-based, the authors have converted the findings to the dollar.
- There were two hospitalizations for neck pain, one from PT and one from the GP group, due to lack of improvement. No cases were hospitalized in the DC group.
- Table 4 on page 4 of the study illustrates the indirect healthcare costs such as absenteeism from work and professional home care.
  - *"Patients treated in the manual therapy group had less work absenteeism and smaller indirect healthcare costs. In addition the number of sessions utilized was lower for the manipulation group than for the physiotherapy groups."*
- Table 5 on page 4 of the study compares direct, indirect, and total costs.
  - *"When comparing the direct, indirect, and total costs, the manual therapy group was statistically significantly lower than the PT and GP groups."*
- Figure 2 on page 5 of the study illustrates head-to-head findings of manual therapy versus physiotherapy cost data.
  - *"Manual therapy compared to physiotherapy was found to be more effective while being less expensive."*
- Figure 3 on page 5 of the study illustrates head-to-head findings of manual therapy versus GP care in terms of cost.
  - *"Manual therapy compared to care by a general practitioner was found to be more effective while being less expensive."*

Potential Questions and Objections

- Not in U.S. dollars.
    - "The authors do convert the values."

Patient Types

- Patients who have a limit in their insurance benefits for PT or chiropractic care
- Patients whose pain is limiting their ability to work

Bottom Line

"Manual therapy is more effective and less costly than PT or GP care for treating neck pain by decreasing the indirect healthcare costs."

"Chiropractic Care of Musculoskeletal Disorders in a Unique Population Within Canadian Community Health Centers." Michael J. Garner, Peter Aker, Jeff Balon, et al. *Journal of Manipulative and Physiological Therapeutics.* 2007;30:165–170.

Proof Source

- Cost-effectiveness for low-income patients on state-funded insurance, making it a good study for audiences with a political focus
- Patient satisfaction
- Safety

Abstract

Objective: This study was part of a larger demonstration project integrating chiropractic care into publicly funded Canadian community health centers. This pre/post study investigated the effectiveness of chiropractic care in reducing pain and disability as well as improving general health status in a unique population of urban, low-income, and multiethnic patients with musculoskeletal (MSK) complaints.

Methods: All patients who presented to one of two community health center–based chiropractic clinics with MSK complaints between August 2004 and December 2005 were recruited to participate in this study. Outcomes were assessed by a general health measure (Short Form-12), a pain scale (VAS), and site-specific disability indexes (Roland-Morris Questionnaire and Neck Disability Index), which were administered before and after a 12-week treatment period.

Results: Three hundred twenty-four patients with MSK conditions were recruited into the study, and 259 (80.0%) of them were followed to the study's conclusion. Clinically important and statistically significant positive changes were observed for all outcomes (Short Form-12: physical composite score mean change = 4.9, 95% confidence interval [CI] = 3.8–6.0; VAS: current pain mean change = 2.3, 95% CI = 1.9–2.6; Neck Disability Index: mean change = 6.8, 95% CI = 5.4–8.1; Roland-Morris Questionnaire: mean change = 4.3, 95% CI = 3.6–5.1). No adverse events were reported.

Conclusions: Patients of low socioeconomic status face barriers to accessing chiropractic services. This study suggests that chiropractic care reduces pain and disability as well as improves general health status in patients with MSK conditions. Further studies using a more robust methodology are needed to investigate the efficacy and cost-effectiveness of introducing chiropractic care into publicly funded health care facilities.

Promotional Strengths

- Published in *JMPT.*
- Recent publication: 2007.
- Large study population: $n = 259$.
- Mixture of authors, including Pran Manga, a prominent Canadian health economist.
- Part of a larger demonstration project that was discussed in Chapter 8.
- Funded by the Ontario Ministry of Health and Long-Term Care.
- Table 1 on page 166 of the study illustrates the patient demographics that represent the low socioeconomic profile.
  - *"Seventy-three percent of the patients were females and 62% of the patients had a household income of less than $19,999, which at the time of the study was just under the $20,337 poverty line. In addition, 83% had chronic pain greater than 3 months duration and 56% had lumbar treatments."*

- Tables 2, 3, and 4 on page 167 of the study recount the efficacy data:
  - *"Patients treated with chiropractic care had clinically important changes in VAS, Disability, and SF-12 and statistically significant changes in VAS, RMQ, and NDI."*
- Patient satisfaction is discussed on page 168 of the study:
  - *"Seventy-eight point eight percent of patients indicated that they were 'very satisfied' with the care and 18.9% were 'satisfied.'"*
- Patient safety is noted on page 169 of the study under the heading of "Description of the Study Sample and Follow-Up": No adverse events were reported or observed.

Potential Questions and Objections

- Promoting this in an upper-class geographic area is not applicable.
- If your practice does not accept Medicaid or state-funded insurance, you are promoting a patient demographic not appropriate for your clinic.
- No control group.
  - *"Most patients receiving care in these settings receive care for conditions that could result in death, not lower back pain. As such, there is no control group because lower back pain does not result in death and is therefore not commonly treated. It is now demonstrated that offering care for LBP could improve disability and reduce work absenteeism."*
- Difficult language barriers.
  - *"Difficult for every healthcare professional."*

Patient Types

- Lower income patients with lower back and neck pain on Medicaid
- Patients with lower socioeconomic barriers to care

Bottom Line

"Patients in lower socioeconomic environments can benefit from chiropractic care by decreasing pain and disability, which may positively affect their ability to work and improve their overall health."

The above study does not examine cost outright; however, the indirect costs do factor in if a patient's disability and pharmacological management could be reduced. In addition, chronic pain can be associated with higher rates of depression and sedentary lifestyles. In this way, treating their back pain can positively impact their overall health.

Conclusion

Many studies address the cost of chiropractic care. Each has its own unique angle that allows for flexibility in your sales presentations as well as the audience you choose to promote to.

It should be more clear than ever the importance of a treat-and-release philosophy. Based on figures from the National Board of Chiropractic Examiners 2005 Annual Survey, it appears as though maintenance or wellness treatments are but a small fraction of a chiropractor's overall business.

Many insurance companies are now focusing on provider report cards for all healthcare professionals. These report cards grade providers against their geographic peers to identify treatments that routinely fall short of or are excessive for the diagnosis. Managed care profiles are defining the chiropractic profession's usefulness in the healthcare arena and therefore shaping all aspects of our standing in managed care facilities as well as at the political level. As more of these managed care reports are made available, it is hoped that chiropractic reimbursement rates and patient accessibility will improve.

REFERENCES

1. Manga P. Economic case for the integration of chiropractic services into the health care system. *J Manipulative Physiol.* 2000; 23(2):118–122.

2. Legorreta AP, Metz RD, Nelson CF, Ray S, Chernicoff HO, Dinubile NA. Comparative analysis of individuals with and without chiropractic coverage: patient characteristics, utilization, and costs. *Arch Intern Med.* 2004;164:1985–1992.

3. American Chiropractic Association. *Utilization, Cost, and Effects of Chiropractic Care on Medicare Program Costs.* July 2001 Executive Summary Available from the ACA at www.acatoday.com.

Chapter 11

The Competition

Introduction to Competitive Selling

For the purposes of promoting chiropractic to the medical profession, *competition* is defined as anything that a doctor might use as a first, second, or third line of therapy for conditions that chiropractic care is equally indicated for. Manipulation has been making its debut appearances in treatment guidelines with increasing frequency. Chiropractors have been passionately defending their primary treatment tool, manipulation, and patiently waiting for the medical world to take note. The good news is they are, both in their own medical journals such as *Spine, Annals of Internal Medicine, New England Journal of Medicine* to name a few, as well as by increasing demand from patients demanding a less invasive treatment approach.

Others in the healthcare industry have taken note as well, such as physical therapists. The response by the physical therapy (PT) industry to the increasing competition not only from the chiropractic industry but to the changing face of health care is a campaign geared toward being recognized as neuromuscular specialists and increasing access and treatment tools (including manipulation) through advanced degrees such as Doctor of Physical Therapy. This is a viable threat to the chiropractic industry.

For too many years the chiropractic profession has protected chiropractic care, which utilizes manipulation as its primary tool. Chiropractors and their associations stand up and react to negative reports and press articles. Our field practitioners continue to hope that some change will come and medical relations and attitudes toward us will become more positive and interactive with all of the positive strides in research and professional advancement. Guess what? The positive evidence has been out long enough to see that this is not what is happening. As such, we can either sit by and watch others utilize our primary tool and become leaders in the treatment of back pain and lose our identity as healthcare providers who specialize in spinal manipulation or we can go out and secure our rightful market share. I am not anti–PT, anti-medicine, anti-acupuncture, anti-naturopath, or anti-massage. I am very much against doing nothing to enhance our standing as healthcare professionals who have a valid service to provide patients with musculoskeletal complaints. It is time to take a stand by educating professionals, and with any selling process there is always a competitor.

The information for chiropractic is evidence based. Any competitor with compelling research that proves a treatment is more efficacious than chiropractic care for the lower back, neck, and headaches—bring it on! Competition doesn't have to be messy and confrontational, but it is competitive and fun when it is done ethically. Finally, before we look at each of the competitors' strengths and weaknesses, it is important to acknowledge the practices that have it right. These are practices that have teamed up and offer a multidisciplinary approach for their patients to choose from. For instance, there is no reason a patient can't have access to medical doctors for medication and diseases of organic nature and under the same roof have access to a physical therapist for exercises, heat, stimulation, and ultrasound, and under the very same roof have access to chiropractic care for manipulation. I have seen these clinics personally, and I commend their forward thinking.

Physical Therapy

The relationship between physical therapists and chiropractors has been almost as tenuous as the one between chiropractors and medical doctors. The exception is for those that have bonded and share office space and co-treat patients. Truly this is a professional relationship so that if the two fields are not working together in multidisciplinary settings, they are fighting it out for medical referrals. Clearly, physical therapists have the lead on medical referrals, but there is room to share some of the marketplace and the evidence illustrates for certain patients that manipulation proves to be extremely efficacious and cost-effective over PT. The advantage that physical therapists have is their already well-established relationship and referral base with medical doctors, and certainly they have enjoyed an open marketplace with no competition, thanks in large part to the disconnect between the medical and chiropractic professions. The disadvantage is the lack of manipulation skills across the PT field and the fact that chiropractors have more hours and training in manipulation. With all the concern about the safety of manipulation, proper training in manipulation cannot be overlooked. Manipulation has the most researched data in the treatment of back pain over any other therapeutic choice, and chiropractors are the recognized professionals that utilize manipulation as their primary treatment tool. Therefore, promoting on efficacy of manipulation is a critical selling point. Chiropractors are not new to manipulation. In fact, manipulation was conceived by chiropractors and, in addition, chiropractors are capable of providing mobilization, massage, heat, ice, traction, exercises, and any other therapeutic treatment that physical therapists offer, provided the state in which they practice allows it. On the flip side, physical therapists are new to manipulation and not all of them are trained to deliver manipulation, although many physical therapists attempt to deliver it despite the fact it is outside of their scope of licensure.

For each of the competitors mentioned in this chapter a SWOT analysis is offered. SWOT stands for strengths, weaknesses, opportunities, and tactics.

Strengths of Physical Therapy

- Readily accepted on insurance plans.
- Readily accepted by medical doctors.
- The American Physical Therapy Association has a well-defined plan to be recognized as the experts in musculoskeletal and neuromuscular function. In addition, physical therapists also promote the restoration of function, improvement of mobility, pain relief, and prevention and tout that they focus on promoting overall fitness and health.
- Trials of conservative physical therapy care for back pain to prevent the need for surgery are routine.
- Physical therapists are experts in many conditions besides back pain, such as stroke rehabilitation, hip fracture, disabilities in newborns, and burn rehabilitation.
- The trend for physical therapists to incorporate spinal manipulation is strengthening. Take one look at the *Journal of Orthopaedic and Sports Physical Therapy* Web site. The entire welcome page is filled with information for integrating spinal manipulation into clinical practice. This is truly an opportunity for identity theft if the chiropractic world allows its primary treatment tool to be introduced, embraced, and welcomed into the medical profession by physical therapists.
  - This journal excerpt examines the use of manipulation by PT students:

    Thrust spinal manipulation was introduced into a physical therapist professional degree curriculum. As part of ongoing student performance monitoring, physical therapy students on their first full-time (8-week) clinical education experience, collected practice pattern and outcome data on individuals with low back complaints. Eight of the 18 first-year students were in outpatient musculoskeletal clinical settings and managed 61 individuals with low back complaints. Patients were seen for an average of 6.2 ± 4.0 visits. Upon initial visit, the student therapists employed spinal manipulation at a rate of 36.2% and spinal mobilization at 58.6%. At the final visit, utilization of manipulation and mobilization decreased (13% and 37.8% respectively), while the utilization of exercise interventions increased, with 75% of patients receiving some form of lumbar stabilization training. Physical therapist students used thrust spinal manipulation at rates that are more consistent with clinical practice guidelines and substantially higher than previously reported by practicing physical therapists."[1]

- Like all healthcare professions, the PT world is embracing evidence-based decision making; thus the incorporation of spinal manipulation.
- Doctor of Physical Therapy Science degrees have been implemented, which are competitive on a portal-of-entry/primary care level with chiropractors.
- PR campaign aimed at reducing costs by advocating "Go to the PT first."[2] An article printed in the *Wall Street Journal* on January 12, 2007, explains the success one local hospital had in significantly decreasing expensive imaging and spine pain–related healthcare costs through using PT first. The success of the plan received nods by Aetna with *increased* reimbursements of $7 per 15 minutes of care as well as nods by major local employers such as Starbucks because of the substantial cost savings. Similar data illustrated in Chapter 8 favor chiropractic care, but the chiropractic industry has had shrinking reimbursements, not increases.
- When advocating conservative care, PT is mentioned, rarely is chiropractic. A case in point is the recent article in *Circulation* on nonsteroidal anti-inflammatory drugs (NSAIDs) that advocates for certain patient populations that the use of NSAIDs should be the last line of defense for chronic pain.[3] Assuming spinal pain, especially in the lumbar region, makes up a significant portion of chronic pain, you would think that chiropractic care would be advocated because the numbers are in our favor for safety. Physical therapy was mentioned as a first line of defense; chiropractic care was notably absent.

Weaknesses of Physical Therapy

- Inconsistent or lack of formal training in manipulation.
- May require preauthorization by a doctor's office.
  - Results in extra unpaid work by the physician.
  - Increased workload on the physician's staff in terms of calls and follow-up.
  - Delayed time in seeking treatment for the patient.
- May take a few days to a couple of weeks to get a first appointment.
- Costs average $140 to $200 for 1 hour of treatment.

- Treatments are longer, which can potentially decrease patient compliance.
- Patients referred to PT don't always follow through with treatment (2 out 6 patients referred made the appointment).[4]

Opportunities to Promote Chiropractic over Physical Therapy

- The evidence-based decision making for spinal manipulation is largely produced by the chiropractic industry, illustrating that chiropractors have a substantial head start in the knowledge and expertise of the daily administration of spinal manipulation. The industry devotes its entire educational curriculum to the management of spinal pain, whereas the PT industry does not. If a doctor is concerned about the safety of spinal manipulation, the safety evidence focuses on qualified and experienced and, most important, licensed chiropractic providers. It is unnerving how many patients report "manipulation" by physical therapists not trained to provide it. When asking patients to describe it, they describe manipulative thrusts, not cracking noises commonly associated with muscle work. Safety of providing manipulation is clearly in favor of chiropractors who have more training and daily experience in thrust spinal manipulation. Evidence-based research on safety is primarily related to chiropractors.
- Patient satisfaction.
- No wait time. Most chiropractors know and sympathize with the negative effect of back pain for patients and accommodate new patients and flare-ups within 24 hours, if not the same day.
- DCs as portal-of-entry care providers require less frequent preauthorizations and treatment approval.
- DC treatment is cost-effective both in direct (medical costs) and indirect costs (loss of work time, home assistance, analgesics).
- Treatment times after the first visit are time effective.
- Basic Medicare patients require a physician's referral and return to see the physician every 30 days to continue with physical therapy, whereas Medicare patients enjoy open access to chiropractic care.

Tactics: Bottom Lined

"When it comes to providing care, chiropractors have a recognized and licensed ability to differentially diagnose mechanical versus nonmechanical back pain and greater experience both in training and daily practice in delivering manipulation. Currently, manipulation has some of the most

extensive research supporting it for the treatment of lower back pain. Chiropractors are more cost-effective than physical therapists."

Proof Sources

- UK BEAM Trial (exercise)[5]
- Haas et al. (MDs provided PT referrals for 25% of the patients; approximate *N* of 231 patients)[6]
- Hoving et al. (exercise)[7]
- Hurwitz et al. (heat and muscle stimulation)[8]
- Bronfort et al. (exercise and ergonomic instruction; PT, home back exercise for low back and PT for neck pain)[9]
- Legorreta et al. (cost)[10]
- Korthals-de Bos et al. (cost)[11]
- UK BEAM Trial (cost)[12]

Medications

One day of watching the news usually provides a summary of the concerns with prescription medication. If a drug isn't being recalled or issued a black box warning, the advertisements list all of the undesired side effects. A black box warning means that medical studies indicate that the drug carries a significant risk of serious or even life-threatening adverse effects. The U.S. Food and Drug Administration (FDA) can require a pharmaceutical company to place a black box warning on the labeling of a prescription drug or in literature describing it. It is the strongest warning that the FDA requires.[13]

Patients are tired of pills that cause side effects and are looking for alternative care to either decrease or eliminate the use of medication altogether. Granted, many conditions do necessitate use of medication either permanently or temporarily, and pharmaceuticals can provide much needed relief to these patients. There are miracle drugs out there and the advancement of health care certainly owes a tremendous amount to the pharmaceutical companies that spend billions of dollars developing these drugs, many of which never make it to the marketplace. Alternatively, it seems that a visit to a doctor's office almost always results in medication being dispensed; NSAIDs are an extremely common prescription and a class of drugs with a black box warning. Specifically, the new black box warnings on NSAIDs are intended to alert doctors and patients to the association of these painkillers with increased risks of heart attacks, ischemic strokes, and gastrointestinal (GI) bleeding.[14] This section provides a SWOT analysis as well as an overview of some of the more common medications used for treating back pain.

Strengths of Medication for Back Pain

- Readily available
- Covered under insurance
- Effective at controlling pain and inflammation

Weaknesses of Medication for Back Pain

- Side effects
  - NSAIDs: GI and cardiovascular are of primary concern
  - Flexeril: Drowsiness
- Safety
  - NSAIDs

Opportunities to Promote Chiropractic over Medication

- Safety and side effects
- Efficacy of manipulation over NSAIDs and muscle relaxants
- Holistic approach that consumers are demanding
- Cost efficacy
- New guidelines for at-risk patients

Should it be mentioned that manipulation has never had a warning issued from the American Heart Association (AHA)? Despite this, public perception is more aware of the misconception of having a stroke with chiropractic manipulation than it is on the dangers of NSAIDs. This report is a must-have in your detail binder because it states the following treatment parameters for the care of musculoskeletal symptoms in patients with or at risk of heart disease and stroke.

"Use of Nonsteroidal Antiinflammatory Drugs: An Update for Clinicians A Scientific Statement from the American Heart Association." Elliott M. Antman, Joel S. Bennett, Alan Daugherty, Curt Furberg, Harold Roberts, Kathryn A. Taubert. *Circulation.* February 26, 2007. Available at http://circ.ahajournals.org.

"Musculoskeletal symptoms should be categorized as those that result from tendonitis/bursitis, those that result from degenerative joint problems (eg, osteoarthritis), or those that result from inflammatory joint problems (eg, rheumatoid arthritis). *Initial treatment should focus on nonpharmacological approaches (eg, physical therapy, heat/cold, orthotics)"[3]* (emphasis added).

Tactics: Bottom Lined

"Chiropractic manipulation is one of the most researched, efficacious, and noninvasive treatment options for patients with lower back pain. The safety of manipulation has been demonstrated time and again and has substantial patient satisfaction. Head-to-head studies against NSAIDs have proven chiropractic to have better efficacy and patient compliance because of fewer dropouts.[15] The AHA is now recommending conservative treatment for patients with or at risk of heart disease or stroke as a first-line defense for musculoskeletal complaints."[15]

Commonly Used Prescriptions for Back Pain

Acetaminophen

Essentially interrupts the patient's perception of pain by disrupting the pain cycle, which decreases pain. Doctors can prescribe it with few precautions as well as prescribe it in combination with other medications. Liver patients (hepatitis, cancer, cirrhosis, etc.) should utilize it with caution.

Seed of Doubt: "Patients with back pain and hepatitis who can't take acetaminophen"

NSAIDs

NSAIDs decrease inflammation and tend to induce fewer GI or ulcer problems than aspirin. There are three types of NSAIDs:

1. Ibuprofen (Advil or Motrin). Effective for muscle type of pain (sprains/strains/overexertion). Patients with active ulcers and those with sensitive stomachs (take with food) should use it cautiously to avoid side effects. It does have blood-thinning properties, and it may interfere with medications for blood pressure and diuretics.

   Seed of Doubt: "Patients with back pain on blood pressure medication who can't take ibuprofen because it will interfere with their blood pressure medications" (Some doctors may feel the interference is negligible.)

2. Naproxen (Aleve). Decreases inflammation and decreases proteins that cause inflammation. Patients who take blood thinners or anticoagulants should avoid this medication due to excessive blood thinning. Patients on monoamine oxidase inhibitors are contraindicated. Patients with sensitive stomachs or ulcers should be cautioned to take it with food.

   Seed of Doubt: "Patients with back pain who may also have GI upset or sensitive stomachs"

3. COX 2 inhibitors (Celebrex; Bextra withdrawn from the market in 2005 due to increased cardiovascular concerns; Vioxx was withdrawn from the market in 2004 for safety reasons). There has been tremendous press about the dangers of NSAIDs. The withdrawal of two out of three branded COX 2 inhibitors certainly reinforces the safety issue surrounding the use of this class of drugs. Although these medications have lower incidences of GI side effects and do not impair blood clotting, they are "safer" to use with patients with ulcers or who may be taking warfarin (Coumadin) and other conditions where bleeding may be a concern. On the flip side, there is the possibility of increased risk of heart attack or stroke. Is it safe to give a patient who is taking Coumadin, an anticoagulant used to prevent the formation of thrombosis, a COX 2 inhibitor even though the drug through other mechanisms can increase the risk of stroke?

   Seed of Doubt: "Patients with back pain who have or are at risk of heart disease and stroke in which case the use of these medications would increase that risk"

Tramadol (Ultram)

This drug is similar to narcotics and changes the way the body perceives pain. Patients who take these are long-term pain sufferers; however, they are frequently used in the acute setting as well. They work similarly to Tylenol but are stronger than acetaminophen and have a smaller narcotic effect. There is not an anti-inflammatory effect. Ultram is utilized to control flare-ups of chronic conditions. There is a real potential risk of serious side effects with overdose and respiratory depression. Caution should be taken if the patient is also taking antidepressant medication or has drug-seeking behavior. It is not recommended for use during pregnancy and can make patients feel spacey. There has been talk about moving this medication into the narcotics category.

   Seed of Doubt: "Patients with chronic pain who are prone to developing addictions for whom this drug may not be a suitable choice"

Narcotics

The next line of defense is the narcotics, which includes Codeine such as Tylenol 3 (weakest), propoxyphene (Darvocet), hydrocodone bitartrate and acetominophen (Vicodin), and oxycodone (Percocet, strongest). Narcotic medications have strong side effects of drowsiness, constipation, and to some degree addiction. It should also be noted that acetaminophen is already included in this package, so concomitant use of acetaminophen is unnecessary. These medications help the patient manage pain through dissociation. The indications for these medications are for 2 weeks or less. Narcotics usually need to be increased over time because tolerance builds up.

> *Seed of Doubt:* "Patients with back pain who can't afford to be drowsy or those with drug-seeking tendencies"

Muscle Relaxants

Muscle relaxants create a sedative effect for muscle spasms associated with back pain. Carisoprodol (Soma) carries a cautionary statement for being habit forming, so it is typically prescribed for shorter periods of time. Cyclobenzaprine (Flexeril) can be used longer, but patients with enlarged prostates should be aware of possible urinary retention, and it can also impair mental and physical function. Diazepam (Valium) is utilized short term due to the potential for habit-forming behavior. It can potentially interfere with sleep and acts as a depressant so that patients suffering from depression should not take it.

> *Seed of Doubt:* "Patients with back pain and depression or drug-seeking behaviors"

Oral Steroids

Steroids may be prescribed for their anti-inflammatory effects. They are non-narcotic and for short-term use due to the side effects and complications associated with long-term usage such as osteoporosis, weight gain, and stomach ulcers. Patients who are diabetic or who have an active infection should not utilize oral steroids. Patients with a long history of steroid use for chronic diseases are contraindicated to manipulation due to concern of osteoporosis.

> *Seed of Doubt:* "Patients who are diabetic or who have stomach ulcers"

Selective Serotonin Reuptake Inhibitors

Selective serotonin reuptake inhibitors are approved for the treatment of depression. Interestingly enough, there is some off-label usage for back pain.

> *Seed of Doubt:* "Patients who already take antidepressants for depression and still have back pain"

Proof Sources

- Rubinstein et al. (benefits outweigh the risks for cervical manipulation)[16]
- Rothwell et al. (safety of cervical manipulation)[17]
- Haneline (safety of cervical manipulation)[18]
- Haldeman (overreporting of cervical manipulation safety in the press)[19]
- Oliphant (safety of lumbar manipulation)[20]
- UK BEAM Trial (efficacy of manipulation compared to exercises)[5]
- Haas (efficacy for chronic and acute lumbar pain with manipulation)[6]
- Nyiendo (efficacy of manipulation over NSAIDs for recurrent back pain)[15]
- Hoiriis et al. (efficacy of manipulation over muscle relaxants for sub-acute pain)[21]
- Hoving et al. (efficacy of manual therapy over PT for neck pain)[7]
- Hurwitz et al. (efficacy of manual therapy and mobilization for neck pain; complication rates are higher for medication)[8]
- Bronfort et al. (efficacy of manipulation and mobilization over PT care, neck and lower back)[9]
- Muller (efficacy of manipulation over medication for chronic spinal pain)[22]
- Duke Evidence Report (efficacy of manipulation over medication and PT for headaches)[23]
- Tuchin (decreased medication usage for migraine patients)[24]
- Legorreta (decreased utilization and reliance on medication)[10]
- Sarnat (cost efficacy of manipulation over medication)[25]

Acupuncture

As chiropractors, we have some knowledge of what acupuncture is and clearly understand that it is an alternative form of treatment for neuromuscular conditions. As you begin to formulate your sales strategies with medical doctors who prefer acupuncture, the following facts about acupuncture should be considered.

What Is Acupuncture?

Acupuncture is a traditional Chinese medicine that dates back about 5,000 years. It is the theory of meridians or energy pathways that carry vital force or energy referred to as *qi* (pronounced chee) that form many pathways and layers between vital organs. These pathways can become altered or congested, and acupuncture helps to reroute the pathways to alleviate pain as well as to reroute the energy to help ailments. In addition to the use of very fine needles inserted along the meridian pathway, for up to 360 different points (the same as acupressure pathways) bundles of smoldering herbs may be placed above the needles as a form of heat therapy. This is known as moxibustion. In addition, laser therapy and muscle stimulation may also be used in connection with the acupuncture procedure.

Mechanism of Action

Western medical experts believe that acupuncture works by triggering chemicals, including pain-killing endorphins and perception-altering neurotransmitters and neuropeptides, that influence the endocrine system, and thus affect mood, energy, and immunity.[26]

Conditions for Which Acupuncture Is Used

It is clear that acupuncture works as a short-time benefit; however, long-term relief is still unclear. It has strong efficacy for nausea, and many patients find relief from nausea associated with chemotherapy, pregnancy, and surgery through acupuncture. Dental pain is also well recognized as an indication, and some dentists are also specialists in dental acupuncture. In addition, arthritis, migraine, menstrual cramps, tension headaches, stroke rehab, asthma, drug addictions, nerve pain, depression, and alcoholism are some of the possible conditions alleviated by acupuncture, and most of these have clinical trials with conflicting findings. Acupuncture treats the whole person or personal constitutions, so treatment plans are very individualized. Treatments usually last for 1 to 12 visits.

Acupuncture is very safe, painless, and has very few side effects. It has some limited availability on managed care. Acupuncture has stood the test of time in the face of Western medicine.

Strengths of Acupuncture

- If a doctor looks to homeopathy or alternative care, acupuncture is highly regarded. Possibly this is because it is so different from allopathic care; perhaps it is because it has been around for centuries. It may also be that chiropractors are more similar to allopathic care than acupuncturists are or the fact that chiropractors have a history of audacious treatment claims that still haunt our public perception today.
- Of all the complementary and alternative (CAM) medicines, acupuncture has the most credibility with medical professionals.

- A substantial body of data shows that acupuncture in the laboratory has measurable and replicable physiologic effects that can begin to offer plausible mechanisms for the presumed actions.[27]
- Safety issues are more obsolete. Whereas chiropractic care is extremely safe, so is acupuncture. Unfortunately, the public perception of "neck cracking" is oversensationalized, whereas no derogatory press has occurred with acupuncture.

Weaknesses of Acupuncture

- Not all states license or have regulations for acupuncture.
- Not always covered on insurance (typical cost is $45–$100). With the strong interest in CAM, this has a strong potential to change; however, there is not any cost-efficacy data for acupuncture in the treatment of lower back pain, neck pain, or headaches.
  - The chiropractic profession has cost savings managed care papers in which claimants with access to chiropractic care had overall fewer costs.
- Some insurances that do cover it require referral from a primary care doctor.
- There have been inconsistent research results, and some studies lack quality study design. Of note is that when it comes to back pain, manipulation performed better than acupuncture.
- In an evidence-based world, the lack of scientific foundation of *qi* is problematic, and some physicians have trouble with the philosophic idea that energy is flowing in meridians that can't be identified anatomically.
- Patients can expect unusual questions about their constitution and *qi*. Tongues are frequently examined and terms such as *fire, wind, cold, damp* imbalances can be expected. Patients may feel uncomfortable.
- Patients may be needle phobic, although it seems there is no pain identified with the actual insertion of needles.
- Side effect: occasional mild transitory depression, anxiety, and fatigue.

Opportunities to Promote Chiropractic over Acupuncture

- The strengths of chiropractic do not overlap with the strengths of acupuncture.
- Research of manipulation for lower back, neck, and headaches.
- Acupuncturists are noted and accepted for pain control and nausea associated with chemotherapy and pregnancy. Although manipulation has impact on pain, it also has impact on disability.
- The long-term efficacy has not been determined for acupuncture, whereas long-term data are available for manipulation.

Tactics: Bottom Lined

"Doctor, acupuncture has great appeal and success for patients with nausea from chemotherapy and pregnancy. Certainly, there is also associated pain control with acupuncture. When it comes to lower back, neck, and headache pain, the body of evidence supports chiropractic care not only for long-term pain control but for disability as well over acupuncture.[22] Furthermore, there is more insurance coverage for chiropractic care at this time."

Proof Sources

- Muller (long-term benefit of manipulation over acupuncture)[22]
- Duke (acupuncture had inconsistent results; manipulation is effective for cervicogenic headaches)[23]
- Any study that examines long-term pain control such as the following:
  - UK BEAM (1 year)[5]
  - Haas (48 months)[6]
- Any study on cost simply because there is no cost analysis and insurance benefits is not as positive for acupuncture compared to chiropractic coverage.

Interesting Fact on Acupuncture

Acupuncture was accepted and grew in the 1970s as a result of improved relations between the United States and China. In the early 1970s, American newspaper reporters covering President Richard Nixon's visit to China wrote about a "miraculous" healing art virtually unknown in the United States. The method immediately stimulated the American imagination. According to the news reports, instead of using chemical anesthetics, Chinese acupuncturists were able to block the pain of surgery using only tiny acupuncture needles inserted into the patient at specific points. Even more astonishing, it was said that these simple acupuncture techniques relieved a wide variety of human illnesses, and had worked reliably for people as their only form of medicine, along with herbs, for thousands of years.

That publicity brought acupuncture into great demand by many Americans, some of them seeking a last resort remedy for serious afflictions. However, at the time, this demand was impossible to meet. There were only a few acupuncturists in the United States, so it took several years for acupuncture colleges to establish themselves in the States and train American acupuncturists. Today it is estimated that 15 million persons each year try acupuncture for the first time. In response to this, more than 60 colleges throughout North America graduate some 1,000 new acupuncturists each year.[26]

Massage

If it is your first inclination to dismiss massage as a competitor because massage therapists are not doctors and are openly available, be aware that there are some recently published studies that conclude the efficacy of massage as a first choice over chiropractic and acupuncture. In addition, most forms of alternative health care are not covered by insurance, so why wouldn't a doctor refer to a massage therapist for back pain, neck pain, and headaches?

Strengths of Massage

- Open access
- Public and medical acceptance of its therapeutic value for back pain
- Research efficacy
- An article published in *Forbes* magazine in June 2007 looked at the trend of massage in health care, and the following points illustrate its strong contention as a competitor:
  - Massage therapists routinely receive referrals from orthopedic surgeons, cardiologists, and physicians.
  - In 2006, 30% of the population seeking massage did so for medical and health reasons.
  - Nine million patients talked about massage with their medical providers in 2006.
  - Managed care coverage doubled from 5% in 2005 to 10% in 2006.
  - In 2006, more hospitals offered massage for conditions such as postpartum lower back pain and stiffness from bedrest. This is a one-third increase in hospitals offering massage in just 2 years.[28]

"A Review of the Evidence for the Effectiveness, Safety, and Cost of Acupuncture, Massage Therapy, and Spinal Manipulation for Back Pain." Daniel C. Cherkin, Karen J. Sherman, Richard A. Deyo, and Paul G. Shekelle. *Annals of Internal Medicine.* 2003;138:898–906.

Abstract

Background: Few treatments for back pain are supported by strong scientific evidence. Conventional treatments, although widely used, have had limited success. Dissatisfied patients have, therefore, turned to complementary and alternative medical therapies and providers for care for back pain.

Purpose: To provide a rigorous and balanced summary of the best available evidence about the effectiveness, safety, and costs of the most popular complementary and alternative medical therapies used to treat back pain.

Data sources: MEDLINE, EMBASE, and the Cochrane Controlled Trials Register.

Study selection: Systematic reviews of randomized, controlled trials (RCTs) that were published since 1995 and that evaluated acupuncture, massage therapy, or spinal manipulation for nonspecific back pain and RCTs published since the reviews were conducted.

Data extraction: Two authors independently extracted data from the reviews (including number of RCTs, type of back pain, quality assessment, and conclusions) and original articles (including type of pain, comparison treatments, sample size, outcomes, follow-up intervals, loss to follow-up, and authors' conclusions).

Data synthesis: Because the quality of the 20 RCTs that evaluated acupuncture was generally poor, the effectiveness of acupuncture for treating acute or chronic back pain is unclear. The three RCTs that evaluated massage reported that this therapy is effective for subacute and chronic back pain. A meta-regression analysis of the results of 26 RCTs evaluating spinal manipulation for acute and chronic back pain reported that spinal manipulation was superior to sham therapies and therapies judged to have no evidence of a benefit but was not superior to effective conventional treatments.

Conclusions: Initial studies have found massage to be effective for persistent back pain. Spinal manipulation has small clinical benefits that are equivalent to those of other commonly used therapies. The effectiveness of acupuncture remains unclear. All of these treatments seem to be relatively safe. Preliminary evidence suggests that massage, but not acupuncture or spinal manipulation, may reduce the costs of care after an initial course of therapy.

- The references section of this paper illustrate that the true head-to-head data comparing manipulation and massage are sparse.
- Cost of care and long-term efficacy data will help to combat this paper.

"Use of a Mechanical Massage Technique in the Treatment of Fibromyalgia: A Preliminary Study." C. Gordon, C. Emiliozzi, and M. Zartarian. *Archives of Physical Medicine and Rehabilitation.* 2006;87(1):145–147.

Abstract

Objective: To investigate how a mechanical massage technique (LPG technique) could contribute to the treatment of fibromyalgia.

Design: Feasibility study.

Setting: A single center.

Participants: Ten women having a preexisting diagnosis of fibromyalgia based on American College of Rheumatology criteria were enrolled.

Intervention: Subjects received a total of 15 sessions of mechanical massage administered by a physical therapist once a week.

Main outcome measures: The Fibromyalgia Impact Questionnaire and a physical examination scoring tender points (number, pain intensity). Evaluations were conducted at the screening visit, after 7 sessions (V7), and after completion of 15 sessions (V15).

Results: Most of the parameters (pain intensity, physical function, number of tender points) showed a significant improvement at V15 compared with screening.

Conclusions: The findings suggest the possibility that the studied intervention might be associated with positive outcomes in women with fibromyalgia and support the need for a controlled clinical trial to determine its efficacy.

- This study illustrates a positive research article for massage as a treatment option for fibromyalgia. It is not a head-to-head study, and neither does it mean that chiropractic services can't also utilize soft tissue therapy for these patients.

- In contrast, chiropractic also has three available fibromyalgia studies. It is important to note that all of these studies are preliminary and a trend toward efficacy may exist, but the results are far from conclusive. The studies showing efficacy from a chiropractic standpoint for fibromyalgia are the following:

"Short- and Long-Term Results of Connective Tissue Manipulation and Combined Ultrasound Therapy in Patients with Fibromyalgia." I. Citak-Karakaya, T. Akbayrak, F. Demirtürk, G. Ekici, and Y. J. Bakar. *Journal of Manipulative and Physiological Therapeutics.* 2006;29(7):524–528.

Abstract

Objective: The aim of the study was to evaluate the short-term and 1-year follow-up results of connective tissue manipulation and combined ultrasound (US) therapy (US and high-voltage pulsed galvanic stimulation) in terms of pain, complaint of nonrestorative sleep, and impact on the functional activities in patients with fibromyalgia (FM).

Methods: This is an observational prospective cohort study of 20 female patients with FM. Intensity of pain, complaint of nonrestorative sleep, and impact of FM on functional activities were evaluated by visual analogue scales. All evaluations were performed before and after 20 sessions of treatment, which included connective tissue manipulation of the back daily, for a total of 20 sessions, and combined US therapy of the upper back region every other session. One-year follow-up evaluations were performed on 14 subjects. Friedman test was used to analyze time-dependent changes.

Results: Statistical analyses revealed that pain intensity, impact of FM on functional activities, and complaints of nonrestorative sleep improved after the treatment program ($P < .05$).

Conclusion: Methods used in this study seemed to be helpful in improving pain intensity, complaints of nonrestorative sleep, and impact on functional activities in patients with FM.

"A Combined Ischemic Compression and Spinal Manipulation in the Treatment of Fibromyalgia: A Preliminary Estimate of Dose and Efficacy." G. Haines, and F. Haines. *Journal of Manipulative and Physiological Therapeutics.* 2000;23(4):225–230.

Abstract

Objectives: To provide preliminary information on whether a regimen of 30 chiropractic treatments that combines ischemic compression and spinal manipulation effectively reduces the intensity of pain, sleep disturbance, and fatigue associated with fibromyalgia. In addition, to study the dose-response relation and identify the baseline characteristics that may serve as predictors of outcome.

Design: Subjects were assessed with self-administered questionnaires taken at baseline, after 15 and 30 treatments, and 1 month after the end of the treatment trial.

Setting: Private practice.

Methods: Participating subjects were adult members of a regional Fibromyalgia Association. Participating subjects had fibromyalgia for more than 3 months. They received 30 treatments including ischemic compression and spinal manipulation. The 3 outcomes being evaluated were pain intensity, fatigue level, and sleep quality. A minimum 50 improvement in pain intensity from baseline to the end of the treatment trial was needed to include the patient in the respondent category.

Results: Fifteen women (mean age 51.1 years) completed the trial. A total of 9 (60%) patients were classified as respondents. A statistically significant lessening of pain intensity and corresponding improvement in quality of sleep and fatigue level were observed after 15 and 30 treatments. After 30 treatments, the respondents showed an average lessening of 77.2 (standard deviation = 12.3) in pain intensity, and an improvement of 63.5 (standard deviation = 31.6) in sleep quality, and 74.8 (standard deviation = 23.1) in fatigue level. The improvement in the 3 outcome measures was maintained after 1 month without treatment. Subjects with less than 35 improvement after 15 treatments did not show a satisfactory response after 30 treatments. A trend, determined as not statistically significant, suggests that older subjects with severe and more chronic pain and a greater number of tender points respond more poorly to treatment.

Conclusion: This study suggests a potential role for chiropractic care in the management of fibromyalgia. A randomized clinical trial should be conducted to test this hypothesis.

"The Effectiveness of Chiropractic Management of Fibromyalgia Patients: A Pilot Study." K. L. Blunt, M. H. Rajwani, and R. C. Guerriero. *Journal of Manipulative and Physiological Therapeutics.* 1997;20(6):389–399.

Abstract

Objective: To demonstrate the effectiveness of chiropractic management for fibromyalgia patients using reported pain levels, cervical and lumbar ranges of motion, strength, flexibility, tender points, myalgic score and perceived functional ability as outcome measures.

Design: A. Preliminary randomized control crossover trial. B. Before and after design.

Patients: Twenty-one rheumatology patients (25–70 yr).

Chiropractic interventions: Treatment consisted of 4 wk of spinal manipulation, soft tissue therapy and passive stretching at the chiropractors' discretion.

Control intervention: Chiropractic management withheld for 4 wk with continuation of prescribed medication.

Main outcome measures: Changes in scores on the Oswestry Pain Disability Index, Neck Disability Index, Visual Analogue Scale, straight leg raise, and lumbar and cervical ranges of motion were observed.

Results: Chiropractic management improved patients' cervical and lumbar ranges of motion, straight leg raise and reported pain levels. These changes were judged to be clinically important within the confines of our sample only.

Conclusions: Further study with a sample size of 81 (for 80% power at alpha < or = .05) is recommended to determine if these findings are generalizable to the target population of fibromyalgia sufferers.

Weaknesses of Massage

- Not all massage therapists have therapeutic training. The ones who are capable of therapeutic massage are commonly located within PT and chiropractic offices or hospitals.
- Massage therapists are educated to understand if a disease state is not compatible with massage therapy; however, they are not licensed to differentiate lower back pain from organic back pain. A medical doctor who is making the referral is trained to know the difference, so this isn't necessarily a selling point, but rather a seed of doubt. It does come into play if the patient is not responding to care and is not referred back into the doctor's office.
- Massage therapy is still an out-of-pocket expense and requires multiple visits. The insurance coverage for massage is growing.

Opportunity to Promote Chiropractic over Massage

- Chiropractors are trained in massage therapy or offer it in their offices.
- Chiropractic services are covered under insurance.

- Chiropractors are trained to differentially diagnose and reevaluate the response to treatment.
- Evidence-based research includes head-to-head studies documenting a more efficacious response to treatment over massage therapy.

Proof Sources

- Hoving[7]
- Hurwitz[8]
- Bronfort[9]
- Duke Evidence Report[23] (specifically the studies listed by Bove[29] and Nilsson[30])
  - Bove
  - Nilsson
- Chiropractic education

Tactics: Bottom Lined

Head-to-head data show a benefit of manipulation over massage not only in efficacy but in costs as well. "Chiropractors have substantially more training in treating back pain, including massage therapy and soft tissue work, and the ability to differentially diagnose back pain from many different causes. Chiropractic services are available under insurance coverage."

Naturopaths

Naturopathy treatment *"may include a broad array of different modalities, including manual therapy, hydrotherapy, herbalism, acupuncture, counseling, environmental medicine, aromatherapy, nutritional counseling, homeopathy, and so on. Practitioners tend to emphasize a holistic approach to patient care."[31]* Naturopathy is based on six principles that include the following:

1. First do no harm.
2. The healing power of nature.
3. Identify and treat the cause.
4. Treat the whole person.
5. The physician as teacher.
6. Prevention.

Strengths of Naturopathy

- Growing in popularity and could gain traction and momentum as alternative care grows.
- Naturopaths are primary care physicians who can prescribe medications (although some states restrict the class and type of medication) and two states restrict their practice entirely.

Weaknesses of Naturopathy

- Weak evidence and difficulty attaining funding for research.
- Every state has different licensing and training requirements. Not all states regulate it all. South Carolina and Tennessee prohibit the practice of naturopathy. The American Association of Naturopathic Physicians (AANP) indicates that licensing is available in 14 states and the District of Columbia.
- Medical doctors are skeptical of naturopathic practices because of their "vitalistic" concepts.
- AANP does not list manipulation as one of its key focuses.
- There are a limited number of naturopaths in practice in the United States.
- Not covered under Medicare, an important selling point for baby boomers.

Opportunities for Promoting Chiropractic over Naturopathy

- Chiropractors are licensed and monitored in every state.
- Chiropractic manipulation has evidence-based research that illustrates efficacy, safety, patient satisfaction, and cost-effectiveness.
- Chiropractic manipulation is covered and available on almost all insurance plans, Medicare, Department of Defense, and workers' compensation.
- In the United States alone, there are more than 60,000 licensed chiropractors.

Tactics: Bottom Lined

Don't address the topic of naturopaths unless a doctor does. If and when naturopathy comes up, the preceding opportunities are all that should be necessary to illustrate the benefits of chiropractic care over naturopathy. Furthermore, there is no research evidence on the success of naturopathy treatment of musculoskeletal disorders that illustrates it to be effective over manipulation or chiropractic care.

Proof Sources

- Any efficacy, safety, cost-effectiveness, or patient satisfaction data
- Any training and licensing information
- Any managed care coverage information

Conclusion

It is important to recognize that all components of health care need to come together to help identify which patients will benefit from which type of care provided by which provider. Alternative treatments play an important role in the future of health care from cost and consumer demand standpoints. With the evidence for chiropractic manipulation secure and growing, allopathic and chiropractic providers need to come together in a team environment for the benefit of administering the best care to patients. There should be no sense of threat between these professions. There is, however, some market share competition between chiropractors and other healthcare professions who are picking up manipulation as a treatment tool. Chiropractors have weathered a very rocky storm, never giving up on the efficacy of manipulation. To have it assumed now by other healthcare providers is fair game, but so is competing for market share. That said, for any chiropractors who may have dual degrees in one of the preceding competitive settings or whose practice has a multidisciplinary setting that includes some of the listed competitors, please don't take this personally. As the movie *Jerry Maguire* coined the phrase "show me the money," I say to any who take offense to the information contained in this chapter, "show me the research"!

REFERENCES

1. Flynn TW, Wainner RS, Fritz JM. Spinal manipulation in physical therapist professional degree education: a model for teaching and integration into clinical practice. *J Orthop Sports Ther.* 2006;36(8)577–587.
2. Fuhrmans V. A novel plan helps hospital wean itself off of pricey tests. *Wall Street Journal,* January 12, 2007.
3. Antman E, Bennett J, Daugherty A, Furberg C, Roberts H, Taubert K. Use of nonsteroidal antiinflammatory drugs. An update for clinicians. A scientific statement from the American Heart Association. *Circulation.* 2007;115(12):1634–1642. Available at http://www.ncbi.nlm.nih.gov/pubmed/17325246. Accessed January 24, 2008.

4. Nyiendo J, Haas M, Goodwin P. Patient characteristics, practice activities, and one-month outcomes for chronic, recurrent low-back pain treated by chiropractors and family medicine physicians: A practice-based feasibility study. *JMPT*. 2000; 23:239–245.

5. UK Back pain Exercise And Manipulation (UK BEAM) Trial Team. UK Back pain Exercise And Manipulation (UK BEAM) randomised trial: Effectiveness of physical treatments for back pain in primary care. *Br Med J*. 2004;329:1377.

6. Haas M, Goldberg B, Aickin M, Ganger B, Attwood M. A practice-based study of patients with acute and chronic low back pain attending primary care and chiropractic physicians: two-week to 48-month follow-up. *J Manipulative Physiol Ther*. 2004; 27:160–169.

7. Hoving J, Koes B, de Vet H, et al. Manual therapy, physical therapy, or continued care by a general practitioner for patients with neck pain; a randomized, controlled trial. *Ann Intern Med*. 2002;136:713–722.

8. Hurwitz E, Morgenstern H, Harber P, Kominski G, Yu F, Adams A. A randomized trial of chiropractic manipulation and mobilization for patients with neck pain: clinical outcomes from the UCLA Neck-Pain Study. *Am J Public Health*. 2002;92:1634–1641.

9. Bronfort G, Haas M, Evans R, Bouter L. Efficacy of spinal manipulation and mobilization for low back pain and neck pain: a systematic review and best evidence synthesis. *Spine*. 2004;335–356.

10. Legorreta AP, Metz RD, Nelson CF, Ray S, Chernicoff HO, Dinubile NA. Comparative analysis of individuals with and without chiropractic coverage: patient characteristics, utilization, and costs. *Arch Intern Med*. 2004;164:1985–1992.

11. Korthals-de Bos I, Hoving J, van Tulder M, et al. Cost effectiveness of physiotherapy, manual therapy and general practitioner care for neck pain; economic evaluation alongside a randomised controlled trial. *Br Med J*. 2003;326:911.

12. UK Back pain Exercise And Manipulation (UK BEAM) Trial Team. United Kingdom Back Pain Exercise and Manipulation Randomised Trial: Cost effectiveness of physical treatments for back pain in primary care. *Br Med J*. 2004;329:1381.

13. Wikipedia.com. Black box warning. Available at http://en.wikipedia.org/wiki/Black_box_warning.

14. Lamb T. Black Box Warning for Celebrex and Other NSAIDs. Drug Injury Watch www.drug-injury.com/druginjurycom/2005/06/blackbox_warnin_1.html

15. Nyiendo J, Haas M, Goodwin P. Patient characteristics, practice activities, and one-month outcomes for chronic, recurrent low-back pain treated by chiropractors and family medicine physicians: a practice-based feasibility study. *J Manipulative Physiol Ther*. 2000;23:239–245.

16. Rubinstein S, Leboeuf-Yde C, Knol D, de Koekkoek T, Pfeifle C, van Tulder M. The benefits outweigh the risks for patients undergoing chiropractic care for neck pain: a prospective, multicenter, cohort study. *J Manipulative Physiol Ther*. 2007;30:408–418.

17. Rothwell D, Bondy S, Williams J, Bousser M. Chiropractic manipulation and stroke: a population-based case-control study. *Stroke*. 2001;32:1054–1060.

18. Haneline MT, Lewkovich G. An analysis of the etiology of cervical artery dissections: 1994–2003. *J Manipulative Physiol Ther*. 2005;28:617–622.

19. Haldeman S, Carey P, Townsend M, Papadopoulos C. Clinical perceptions of the risk of vertebral artery dissection after cervical manipulation: The effect of referral bias. *Spine*. 2002;2:334–342.

20. Oliphant D. Safety of spinal manipulation in the treatment of lumbar disk herniations: a systematic review and risk assessment. *J Manipulative Physiol Ther*. 2004; 27:197–210.

21. Hoiriis K, Pfleger B, McDuffie F, et al. A randomized clinical trial comparing chiropractic adjustments to muscle relaxants for subacute low back pain. *J Manipulative Physiol Ther*. 2004;27:388–398.

22. Muller R, Giles L. Long-term follow-up of a randomized clinical trial assessing the efficacy of medication, acupuncture, and spinal manipulation for chronic mechanical spinal pain syndromes. *J Manipulative Physiol Ther*. 2005;28:3–11.

23. McCrory D, Penzien D, Hasselblad V, Gray R. Des Moines, Iowa: Evidence Report: Behavioral and Physical Treatments for Tension-type and Cervicogenic Headache. Duke University Evidence-based Practice Center. Foundation for Chiropractic Education and Research; 2001 Product No.: 2085.

24. Tuchin P, Pollard H, Bonello R. A randomized controlled trial of chiropractic spinal manipulative therapy for migraine. *J Manipulative Physiol Ther*. 2000;23:91–95.

25. Sarnat R, Winterstein J, Cambron J. Clinical utilization and cost outcomes from an integrative medicine independent physician association: An additional 3 year update. *J Manipulative Physiol Ther*. 2007;30:263–269.

26. Pelletier K. *The Best Alternative Medicine*. New York, NY: Simon and Schuster; 2000.

27. Kaptchuk T. Acupuncture: theory, efficacy, and practice. *Ann Intern Med*. 2002; 136:374–383.

28. Van Dusen A. Patients kneading away health ills with massage. More are recognizing that a good rubdown can help with medical issues. Forbes.com. June 15, 2007. Available at http://www.msnbc.msn.com/id/19190927/. Accessed January 24, 2008.

29. Bove G, Nilsson N. Spinal manipulation in the treatment of episodic tension-type headache: A randomized controlled trial. *JAMA*. 1998;280(18):1576–1579.

30. Nilsson N, Christensen LHW, Hartvigsen, J. The effect of spinal manipulation in the treatment of cervicogenic headache. *J Manipulative Physiol Ther*. 1997;20(5):326–330.

31. Wikipedia.com. Naturopathic medicine. Available at http://en.wikipedia.org/wiki/Naturopathic_medicine

Chapter 12

Other Promotional Opportunities

A side from promoting to medical doctors, the sales process and associated research presented in this text can be applied successfully in other situations, most notably to employers and politicians. In addition, knowing evidence-based research will help you secure employment and opens the doors for new public relations.

Promoting to Employers

Back injuries are one of the most costly injuries for medical claims and disability. Chiropractors, being specialists in the treatment and the prevention of lower back and neck injuries, have a service they can provide to employers.

Big-box employers such as Target, Wal-Mart, and grocery stores are interested in curtailing costs. Ways in which chiropractors can help are as follows:

- On-site inspections: Offer to do sporadic on-site visits to observe for:

    Watching for improper lifting

    Inspecting for work hazards

- Work shift change presentations (consisting of a 5-minute or more presentation and could be tied in with on-site inspections)

    Ergonomic lessons

    Proper lifting techniques

    Avoiding workplace injuries

    Proper stretching

- Primary workers' compensation doctor for "nonbleeding disorders" (If a patient is not bleeding, has not suffered an obvious fracture, has not been exposed to chemical substances, and is conscious, employers should send them to your office to reduce medical costs and disability.

Most injuries are musculoskeletal, and you can make any necessary referrals especially if you have medical relationships.

Efficacy

Cost-efficacy

Reduced disability

Work modification programs (Get to know the employer's job positions and physical requirements so that you can place the employee in another job position and not on disability.)

- Other services

Pre and post urinalysis drug screen

Cost is obviously an important issue to employers. Providing cost-effective care and limiting time off of work decreases employers workers' compensation liabilities. Several notable workers' compensation studies have been conducted specifically on chiropractic and the costs of managing workers' compensation claims. Two of the most recent were conducted by the states of Texas and Florida.

"Chiropractic Care of Florida Workers' Compensation Claimants: Access, Costs, and Administration Outcome Trends from 1994–1999." MGT of America. *Topics of Clinical Chiropractic.* 2002; 9(4):33–53.

The authors' conclusions were strongly in favor of chiropractic services for reducing costs and disability:

- "A higher proportion of professional services provided by DCs with specific cases (low back and other musculoskeletal) correlated with lower medical and other claims costs."[1]

- "A higher proportion of professional services provided by DCs with specific cases (low back and other musculoskeletal) correlated with reduced time to reach maximal medical improvement."[1]

- "A higher proportion of professional services provided by DCs with specific cases (specific low back and other musculoskeletal) correlated with shorter return-to-work durations."[1]

"Chiropractic Treatment of Workers' Compensation Claimants in the State of Texas." MGT of America for the Texas Chiropractic Association. 2003.

To order: Contact the Texas Chiropractic Association at (512) 477-9292 or via email: info@chirotexas.org.

The study examined workers' compensation claims from 1996 to 2001 and found that not only was chiropractic care not responsible for the rising workers' compensation claims in the state of Texas, but in fact, "Chiropractic care is associated with lower medical costs and more rapid recovery in the overwhelming majority of studies concerning chiropractic care and workers' compensation costs. . . . The average claim for a worker with a low-back injury was $15,884. However, if a worker received at least 75 percent of his or her care from a chiropractor, the total cost per claimant decreased by nearly one-fourth to $12,202. If the chiropractor provided at least 90 percent of the care, the average cost declined by more than 50 percent, to $7,632."[2]

These two titles are recent and illustrate not only cost but disability. Disability immediately affects an employer financially. Limiting or preventing disability with work modification plans where available will be most appealing to many employers.

Political Lobbying

The chiropractic profession needs your help to ensure that there is a future for chiropractic in health care. You can make an impact politically with your local and state elected officials by utilizing the research and selling style included in this text. Senior/Medicare health care will no doubt be an important issue for any elected official as will health care that provides an alternative to medication and surgery.

The efficacy of manipulation for musculoskeletal conditions and the American Chiropractic Association (ACA) Report for Medicare (reviewed in Chapter 10) will surely be compelling evidence for any political leader. Educating these leaders on the evidence supporting chiropractic can aid in understanding and support for manipulation. How it translates into what it means for their constituents is the key selling point for a politician. If their constituents want it, so do they if they want to be reelected. Safe alternatives to medication and surgery, alternative care providers, and cost-effective health care are all trendy topics in today's world.

The ACA is clearly the chiropractic industry's leader in fighting the political cause. Recently, the ACA sponsored a TeleSeminar titled Lobbying 101. The presenters were Steve Perman, DC, DACBSP, DACBN, and ACA National Legislative Commission member, ACA Alternate Delegate, South Florida, Officer at Large, ACA-PAC Board Chairman, BAC-PAC. The other was John Falardeau, ACA vice president, Government Relations, ACA-PAC. Their presentation is available for purchase as an audio CD by contacting the ACA.

In their presentation, the purposes of lobbying as well as how you can relate the profession's issues to benefits for politicians' constituencies are covered. A few reasons the speakers provided for the purpose of lobbying is to encourage politician support of bills, request proper implementation of existing law, and explain how chiropractic issues can benefit constituents.

The next obvious question is, who are the politicians' constituents? If your geographic area has a Veterans Administration (VA) hospital or large military population, your lobbying might involve requesting proper implementation of existing law, in this case the addition of chiropractors to staff so that veterans and military personnel can access chiropractic benefits.

The elderly population is important in every geographic area. Not only will the evidence on safety be important, but the Medicare Report will be a huge promotional benefit in documenting the cost-effectiveness of chiropractic care. The large baby boomer population can benefit from this as well, and the facts are that seniors are concerned about affordable and noninvasive health care.

Cost-management and cost-efficacy data are important for workers' compensation and high cost of living demographics. You can adapt the research and selling technique in this book to your audience based on how chiropractic services can meet their *needs*.

Creating consumer demand, educating medical doctors, and creating political demand could make a profound impact on our profession's standing and transport us from being outcasts to leaders as musculoskeletal specialists in the healthcare arena.

Employment

Already there has been tremendous positive forward motion. The inclusion of chiropractic in the Department of Defense (DOD) is a major milestone; however, implementation needs to be enforced at the ground level. Aside from being a benefit for DOD patients, it is a benefit for chiropractors to have the opportunity for employment. Major medical group practices with a diverse approach to treatment conditions will be the most likely candidates to consider employing chiropractors. An example is a large physical therapy center that houses physical therapists, medical physicians including osteopaths, and also chiropractors. A second example is large clinics of neurologists that house physiatrists and physical therapists, where it makes sense that a chiropractor would add a solid therapeutic option for patients. Keep in mind that you may need to approach them. Both of these examples are in existence and becoming more common!

The administrative staff that does the hiring must also be educated on how to implement chiropractic services for their patients. That you can provide current evidence-based research on chiropractic manipulation in an educational manner establishes your credibility as well as that of your profession.

By knowing your evidence, you imply trust in your services as an employee and aid in a smooth transition with other healthcare providers.

Job postings for chiropractors can be searched for on the VA Web site at www.va.gov. If you live near a VA hospital, it would behoove you to get to know the local hiring staff or contracting authorities. The DOD is required to add chiropractic staff in the next few years, so introducing yourself now will help you in the future with job placement. Facilities will be listing job or contracting opportunities. Having a jump on the competition and knowing the administration might be tricky, but it will certainly benefit you in the long run. According to Sara J. McVicker, clinical program manager, Primary Care, Patient Care Services (retired) U.S. Department of Veterans Affairs, soldiers are returning from the war with musculoskeletal complaints from carrying heavy gear and jostling in humvees and Bradleys. In addition, she notes that the chiropractors that are currently employed or contracted to provide chiropractic services are often "booked solid or overbooked for acute care needs" from the demand. Furthermore, she notes that 40% of complaints are musculoskeletal, many of which are treatable by chiropractors. By visiting the ACA Web site, members will have access to Sara McVicker's and other keynote speakers' topics for the 2007 National Chiropractic Legislative Conference (NCLC) conference. I strongly recommend listening to all of them for additional insight into these political and governmental issues.

Public Relations

There are many opportunities to provide a public service for your community, your patients, and medical doctors' patients. Recently, I had an opportunity to sit in on such a service provided to the community by a medical group. At this particular meeting, the discussion was on golf and lower back pain. The medical group had paid a reasonable fee to a local well-known golf pro to come and talk. The first portion of the talk was on back pain, symptoms, and conditions. The second talk was done by the golf pro in which he outlined the proper swing technique and the errors that could lead to back pain, either acute or chronic.

Chiropractors have the ability to offer this same type of service and can utilize doctors' waiting rooms and employer contacts to promote these services to medical patients and employees. Medical doctors could also be asked to participate to provide a cohesive healthcare team approach with information on medications, and other options for back pain.

Opportunities such as these are endless when we have the ability to work in conjunction with a variety of different healthcare providers and therefore access different perspectives and treatment options. Opening your facility to provide the space for these kinds of talks provides you the opportunity to provide education on back pain and begin the process of gaining recognition as a specialist in your community. Providing light snacks and drinks is a nice touch. Your literature should indicate who will be speaking, the time frame, and a map to your facility. Providing a press release for a free healthcare talk to your local newspapers and news stations will increase the attendance, but make sure you contact the newspapers to see how far in advance they need to publish your release. Typically you will contact the "health" editor.

Chiropractors and medical doctors have a multitude of topics to present together, but it takes a relationship with a medical physician to begin these multidisciplinary healthcare talks.

Samples

In pharmaceuticals, one of the best tools for feedback was the ability to give samples to doctors. It required their signature and therefore provided an almost guaranteed opportunity to talk to doctors. That option does not exist for chiropractors; however, the opportunity to check in and gain some sales information does still exist. We just have to think outside the box.

One solution that presents itself is the opportunity to provide a tester product such as Biofreeze samples or any other sample that you like. Not only does it reinforce the musculoskeletal focus of our care but it provides a goodwill service for doctors' patients. It also provides you with an opportunity to check in with the doctor as well as gain insight into the practice's habits. For example, if you provide samples for the doctor, you can and should place a sticker that indicates "courtesy of" and your name or practice name. If you place it in the doctor's samples closet, which would be acceptable for most practices, you should place it next to an analgesic sample such as Celebrex or next to a skeletal muscle relaxant such as Flexoril. The fact that you are able to see the medications that the doctor utilizes will give you insight into which medications you should know inside and out, in other words, what advantages does your service offer that the medications don't.

Additionally, these promotional products allow you an opportunity to visit the office more often, which provides you with a circumstance to initiate more consistent contact with the doctor, even if it is just to say hello. A few cautions to be aware of are the following:

- You aren't there to be a pharmaceutical rep. Those samples are a courtesy provided by your office in honor of a mainstream working relationship.
- These products cost you money. They shouldn't be expected. If the doctor's practice calls on a consistent basis to tell you they've run out of sam-

ples, it could be a problem that could put you in an awkward circumstance. Providing the practice with the name and number so that they can get their own samples could be enough to casually end the expectation that you are supposed to provide the samples. Explaining to the staff and doctor that you are personally paying for these samples should also suffice. If you are getting a ton of referrals, you might consider the cost and time to supply these samples worth it. As with luncheons and dinners, providing samples is not a necessary step, just an option.

Web Site Marketing

Patients today are savvy consumers. The Internet has certainly made sure of that. Marketing your services on a Web site won't necessarily provide you with an immediate source of new patients, but it could be a phenomenal way to market to your existing patients. Providing patients with access to your Web site allows you to post up-to-date research, information on public outreach events, and monthly preventative issues. Patients like to research their own conditions, so why not provide them a Web site to research their back pain from a chiropractic perspective as well as providing links to the Foundation for Chiropractic Education and Research, the ACA, and more?

By opening the door to medical offices, we open up more than just patient referrals: We open up lasting professional relationships and more opportunity for positive public relations. Practicing in relative isolation no longer applies.

Conclusion

Evidence-based health care is here to stay. Not only should you be familiar with it to provide the most comprehensive and up-to-date care for your patients, but you also should take advantage of it as a tool to finally break through barriers with the medical community and therefore with their patients. Not only are there financial benefits through new patient referrals, but by minimizing costly advertising they also extend to establish credibility in the healthcare community and to maintain our viability as specialists in manipulation before our competition does it for us.

As you have seen in this text, there are many ways to present a study. As you become familiar with the research, you may find other portions of the study to promote. This text is not meant to be rigid but rather to offer you insight and ideas on how to best promote your practice to the medical community. It can be flexible to meet your budget information needs. As long as you stick to evidence-based health care, your promotions will be legitimate and well received by the medical community.

I wish you the best of luck and invite you to contact me with questions, comments, success stories, and troubleshooting questions.

Good Selling!

Christina Acampora
Christina.acampora@alignedmethods.com

REFERENCES

1. MGT of America. "Chiropractic care of Florida workers' compensation claimants: access, costs, and administration outcome trends from 1994–1999." *Topics of Clinical Chiropractic*. 2002;9(4):33–53.

2. MGT of America. "Chiropractic treatment of workers' compensation claimants in the state of Texas." Texas Chiropractic Association, 2003.

3. American Chiropractic Association. Utilization, Cost, and Effects of Chiropractic Care on Medicare Program Costs. July 2001. Executive summary available from the ACA. www.acatoday.com

Companies with Promotional Products

Aligned Methods (http://www.alignedmethods.com/)

Aligned Methods was founded by this book's author, Christina Acampora, DC. It is the only company solely dedicated to bridging the gap between the medical and chiropractic communities. As an industry leader providing affordable promotional materials to chiropractic physicians, Aligned Methods dedicates itself to working with national, state, and local chiropractic communities to positively affect the public image and acceptance within the medical communities of chiropractic care. Aligned Methods provides both products and membership services.

Master Visual Aids

A large variety of master visual aids (MVAs) is available for all phases of the promotional process, and new MVAs are promptly produced as new research is published. MVAs illustrating efficacy, safety, and cost are available from a variety of research articles including but not limited to the following topics:

- Overview of chiropractic care including the mechanism of action of spinal manipulation
- Lumbar research for manipulation
- Cervical research for manipulation
- Headache research for manipulation
- Safety of spinal manipulation
- Cost-effectiveness of chiropractic care
- Patient satisfaction with chiropractic care

Membership Services

Aligned Methods is dedicated to keeping chiropractors informed of the latest promotional research while also keeping them abreast of the competition.

We understand that your time is limited, so we do the research for you and continually post new research summaries that would be appropriate to use from a promotional perspective. Careful monitoring of applicable research journals including the competition ensures members that they are up to date and current in their promotional efforts.

- In addition to keeping up with the latest research, membership entitles you to use a variety of chat boards that address current promotional activities, legalities, and research. Members have full access to common objections by medical professionals and how they have been successfully handled by other chiropractors.
- Public relations efforts that illustrate joint presentations with medical physicians are posted along with a plan of implementation.
- There are many more benefits to membership:
  - Monthly e-letters.
  - Promotional efforts related to employers and political figures.
  - E-mail promotional support. Have a specific question that isn't answered in the chat boards? If so, Dr. Acampora will personally answer the question for you.

Aligned Methods is committed to providing chiropractors with the best promotional products with a strong commitment to service and affordability. Visit us today to learn more.

American Chiropractic Association (http://www.acatoday.com/)

The ACA has long been a leader in providing promotional products for chiropractors. It has several products that help chiropractors promote to the medical and employment communities. The ACA is the leader in the political efforts for the chiropractic industry. Visit the Web site to view products.

Foundation for Chiropractic Education and Research (http://www.fcer.org/)

Aside from being the leader in chiropractic research, FCER also offers promotional products that could be used to aid the chiropractic physician in a promotional setting. Visit the Web site to view products.

Web Site Resources

Federal

Clinical Trials

Agency for Healthcare Resources and Quality (http://www.ahcpr.gov)

American Public Health Association, Chiropractic Healthcare Section (http://www.apha-chc.org/)

Health Resources and Services Administration (http//www.hrsa.gov/)

National Center for Complementary and Alternative Medicine (http://nccam.nih.gov/)

National Guideline Clearinghouse (http//www.guideline.gov/)

National Institutes of Health (http://www.nih.gov/)

National Institutes of Health Clinicaltrials.gov (http://www.clinicaltrials.gov/)

U.S. Department of Health and Human Services (http://www.os.dhhs.gov/)

U.S. Department of Veterans Affairs (http://www.va.gov/)

Chiropractic

Academy of Chiropractic Orthopedists (http//www.dcorthoacademy.com/)

American Chiropractic Association (http//www.acatoday.com/)

American Chiropractic College of Radiology (http//www.accr.org/)

American College of Chiropractic Orthopedists (http//www.accoweb.org/)

Association of Chiropractic Colleges (http//www.chirocolleges.org/)

Canadian Chiropractic Association (http//www.ccachiro.org/)

Chiropractic Economics (http//www.chiroeco.com/)

The Chiropractic Report (http//chiropracticreport.com/tcr/home.htm)

College on Forensic Sciences (http//www.forensic-sciences.org/)

Congress of Chiropractic State Associations (http//www.cocsa.org/)

The Council on Chiropractic Education (http//www.cce-usa.org/)

Federation of Chiropractic Licensing Boards (http//www.fclb.org/)

Immunization Information Resource (http//www.apha-chc.org/
vaccinfo/default.htm)

Institute of Evidence-Based Chiropractic (http//www.chiroevidence.com/)

International Board of Chiropractic Examiners (http//www.ibce.org/)

International Chiropractors Association (http//www.chiropractic.org/)

Journal of Manipulative and Physiological Therapeutics
(http//www.journals.elsevierhealth.com/periodicals/ymmt/claim)

National Board of Chiropractic Examiners (http//www.nbce.org/)

World Chiropractic Alliance (http//www.worldchiropracticalliance.org/)

World Federation of Chiropractic (http//www.wfc.org/)

Chiropractic College Links

Cleveland Chiropractic College (www.clevelandchiropractic.edu)

Life Chiropractic College West (www.lifewest.edu)

Life University School of Chiropractic (www.life.edu)

Logan College of Chiropractic (www.logan.edu)

National University of Health Sciences (www.nuhs.edu)

New York Chiropractic College (www.nycc.edu)

Northwestern Health Sciences University (www.nwhealth.edu)

Palmer College of Chiropractic (www.palmer.edu)

Parker College of Chiropractic (www.parkercc.edu)

Sherman College of Straight Chiropractic (www.sherman.edu)

Southern California University of Health Sciences (www.scuhs.edu)

Texas Chiropractic College (www.txchiro.edu)

University of Bridgeport College of Chiropractic
(www.bridgeport.edu/chiro/)

Western States Chiropractic College (www.wschiro.edu)

Chiropractic Research Web Sites

Aligned Methods (http://www.alignedmethods.com/)

American Chiropractic Association (http://www.acatoday.com/)

Australia Spine Research Association (http://www.spinalresearch.com.au/)

The Bone and Joint Decade 2000–2010 Task Force on Neck Pain and Its Associated Disorders (http://www.nptf.ualberta.ca/)

CAM on PubMed (http://www.nlm.nih.gov/nccam/camonpubmed/)

Chiropractic and Health (http://www.chiropracticresearch.org/)

The Chiropractic Report (http://www.chiropracticreport.com/)

Chiropractic Research (http://www.chiro.org/)

The Cochrane Library (http://www.thecochranelibrary.org)

Council on Chiropractic Guidelines and Practice Parameters (http://www.ccgpp.org/)

Foundation for Chiropractic Education and Research (http://www.fcer.org)

Institute of Evidence-Based Chiropractic (http://www.chiroevidence.com/)

Journal of Chiropractic Education (http://www.journalchiroed.com/)

Manual Alternative and Natural Therapy Index System (http://www.healthindex.com)

New York Chiropractic College (www.nycc.edu)

Northwestern Health Sciences University (http://www.nwhealth.edu/)

Palmer College of Chiropractic (http://www.palmer.edu/)

PubMed (http://www.pubmed.com/)

To Your Health (http://www.chiropracticresearchreview.com/)

Common Research Search Phrases

cervical	headache
neck	orthopedic
chiropractic	randomized controlled trials
neck pain	comparative study
patient satisfaction	review literature
manipulation	osteopathy medicine

Other Helpful Web Sites

American Academy of Pain Management (http://www.aapainmanage.org/)

American Academy of Spine Physicians (http://www.spinephysicians.org/)

Competitive Organizations

American Association of Acupuncture and Oriental Medicine
(http://www.aaom.org/)

American Massage Therapy Association (http://www.amtamassage.org/)

American Medical Massage Association
(http://www.americanmedicalmassage.com/)

American Naturopathic Medical Association (http://www.anma.com/)

American Osteopathic Association (http://www.osteopathic.org/)

American Physical Therapy Association (http://www.apta.org/)

General Medication Web Sites

http://www.drug-injury.com/

http://www.drugs.com/

http://www.fda.gov/

http://www.rxlist.com/

http://www.medicinenet.com/

http://www.safemedication.com/

http://www.nlm.nih.gov/medlineplus

General Safety Statistics

Reported Activities Involving the Cervical Spine Suspected of Being Involved with Disruption of Cerebral Circulation

Athletics

Dental work

Overhead work

Self-manipulation

Spontaneous vertebral artery dissection

Backing up a car

Hair dressing

Postural head changes

Spinal manipulation

Traction and short-wave diathermy[1]

Estimated Rate of Strokes from Manipulation

Cervical spinal manipulation[2,3]	1 in 1.7 million procedures
Cervical spinal manipulation[2,4]	1 in 2 million procedures

REFERENCES

1. Rome PL. Perspective: an overview of comparative considerations of cerebrovascular accidents. *Chiropractic J Australia.* 1999;23(3):87–102.
2. Rosner A. Spontaneous cervical artery dissections and implications for homocysteine. *J Manipulative Physiol Ther.* 2004;27:124–132.

3. Haldeman S, Carey P, Townsend M, Papadopoulos C. Arterial dissections following cervical manipulation: the chiropractic experience. *Can Med Assoc J.* 2001;165:905–906.

4. Terrett AGJ. *Current Concepts in Vertebrobasilar Complications Following Spinal Manipulation.* West Des Moines, IA: NCMIC Group, Inc.; 2001.

Chiropractic Degree and Educational Background

What Is a Chiropractic Degree in Relation to Other Healthcare Degrees?

First-professional degree in chiropractic (DC) is a program that prepares individuals for the independent professional practice of chiropractic, a healthcare and healing system based on the application of noninvasive treatments and spinal adjustments to alleviate health problems caused by vertebral misalignments affecting bodily function as derived from the philosophy of Daniel Palmer. This program includes instruction in the basic medical sciences, chiropractic theory and science, postural and spinal analysis, diagnostic radiology and ultrasound, adjustment technique, patient counseling, professional standards and ethics, and practice management.[1]

REFERENCE

1. Universities.com. First-Professional degree in Chiropractic. Available at http://www.universities.com/On-Campus/FirstProfessional_degree_Health_Professions_and_Related_Clinical_Sciences_Chiropractic_DC_DCM.html. Accessed January 24, 2008.

Samples of First-Professional Degrees

- Doctor of Chiropractic (DC or DCM)
- Doctor of Dental Surgery (DDS) or Doctor of Dental Medicine (DMD), depending on the individual school attended
- Doctor of Osteopathic Medicine (DO)
- Doctor of Optometry (OD)
- Doctor of Medicine (MD)
- Doctor of Pharmacy (PharmD)
- Doctor of Podiatric Medicine (DPM)
- Doctor of Psychology (PsyD)

Chiropractic Education

Chiropractic Education in Terms of Average Hours of Lectures, Laboratories, and Clinics in 16 Chiropractic Colleges

		Chiropractic Schools	
Variable	Total	Basic Science	Clinical Science
Lecture hours	2,675	1,020	1,655
Laboratory hours	1,115	400	715
Clinical hours	1,010	0	1,010
Total	4,800	1,420	3,380

Source: Center for Studies in Health Policy, Inc., Washington, DC. Personal communication of 1995 unpublished data from Meredith Gonyea, PhD. Available at http://www.chiroweb.com/archives/ahcpr/chapter3.htm.

Average Total Contact Hours in Specific Clinical Subjects Taught in 16 Chiropractic Colleges (includes lectures and laboratories)

Clinical Subject	Hours	% of Total
Adjustive technique/spinal analysis	555	22%
Physical/clinical/laboratory diagnosis	410	17%
Diagnostic imaging, radiology	305	12%
Principles of chiropractic	245	10%
Orthopedics	135	6%
Physiologic therapeutics	120	5%
Nutrition/dietetics	90	4%
Professional practice and ethics	65	3%
Biomechanics	65	3%
Gynecology/obstetrics	55	2%
Psychology	55	2%
Research methods	50	2%
Clinical pediatrics and geriatrics	50	2%

(continues)

*Average Total Contact Hours in Specific Clinical Subjects Taught in
16 Chiropractic Colleges (includes lectures and laboratories) (continued)*

Clinical Subject	Hours	% of Total
First aid and emergency	45	2%
Dermatology	30	1%
Otolaryngology	25	1%
Other	160	7%
Total hours of clinical training	2,460	100%

Source: Center for Studies in Health Policy, Inc., Washington, DC. Personal communication of 1995 unpublished data from Meredith Gonyea, PhD. Available at http://www.chiroweb.com/archives/ahcpr/chapter3.htm.

*Comparisons of the Overall Curriculum Structure for Chiropractic and
Medical Schools*

	Chiropractic Schools		Medical Schools	
	Mean	Percentage	Mean	Percentage
Total contact hours	4,822	100%	4,667	100%
Basic science hours	1,416	29%	1,200	26%
Clinical science hours	3,406	71%	3,467	74%
Chiropractic science hours	1,975	41%	0	0
Clerkship hours	1,405	29%	3,467	74%

Source: Center for Studies in Health Policy, Inc., Washington, DC. Personal communication of 1995 unpublished data from Meredith Gonyea, PhD. Available at http://www.chiroweb.com/archives/ahcpr/chapter3.htm.

*Comparison of Hours of Basic Sciences Education in Medical and
Chiropractic Schools*

	Chiropractic Schools		Medical Schools	
Subject	Hours	% of Total	Hours	% of Total
Anatomy	570	40	368	31
Biochemistry	150	11	120	10
Microbiology	120	8	120	10
Public health	70	5	289	24
Physiology	305	21	142	12
Pathology	205	14	162	14
Total Hours	**1,420**	**100**	**1,200**	**100**

Source: Center for Studies in Health Policy, Inc., Washington, DC. Personal communication of 1995 unpublished data from Meredith Gonyea, PhD. Available at http://www.chiroweb.com/archives/ahcpr/chapter3.htm.

Questionnaires to Include in a Detail Binder

The following objective measurement forms would be an ideal addition to your detail binder. An Internet search will provide you with multiple sites to download the individual questionnaires that in most cases are free.

- Roland Morris Questionnaire
- Short Form McGill Pain Questionnaire and Pain Diagram
- Revised Oswestry Low Back Disability Index
- Neck Disability Index
- Headache Disability Inventory
- RAND 36-Item Health Survey Instrument

Ongoing Research Projects

The following low back and cervical studies are copied directly from Clinical Trials.gov. As it states on its Web site, ClinicalTrials.gov is a registry of federally and privately supported clinical trials conducted in the United States and around the world. ClinicalTrials.gov gives you information about a trial's purpose, who may participate, locations, and phone numbers for more details. Not only does this Web site provide the reader with a look at upcoming research, but it also illustrates potential competitive research as well as other potential treatments for conditions ranging from magnet therapy to surgery. To access information visit http://clinicaltrials.gov, click List by Condition tab, and then click Symptoms and General Pathology. Then, select low back or neck pain or headache.

This Web site does not provide any information on the findings of the studies or which publication they may be published in or if they will even be published. It does, however, list the institution that is sponsoring the study; a visit to the institution's Web site can yield more information. It is quite possible that some of these studies, especially those marked as completed, will be published between the writing and the actual release of this text. The important research search parameters when watching for these studies' appearance in the literature will be the interventions and conditions that they list for each trial.

Low Back Studies

One hundred sixty-one studies were listed in this category in December 2007. The following have a chiropractic focus:

7 Active, not recruiting	**Spinal Manipulative Therapy for Low Back Pain** Condition: Low back pain Intervention: Procedure: manipulative therapy

**8 Active,
not recruiting**

Chiropractic and Exercise for Seniors with Low Back Pain
Condition: Low back pain
Interventions: Procedure: Chiropractic manual treatment + home exercise (procedure + behavior);
Procedure: Supervised rehabilitative exercise + home exercise;
Behavioral: Home exercise

22 Completed

Physical CAM Therapies for Chronic Low Back Pain
Condition: Chronic low back pain
Interventions: Procedure: massage therapy;
Procedure: chiropractic;
Procedure: acupuncture

41 Completed

Manipulation, Exercise, and Self-Care for Low Back Pain
Condition: Low back pain
Interventions: Procedure: Chiropractic spinal manipulation;
Procedure: Exercise; Behavioral: Self-care

54 Completed

Usual Care versus Choice of Alternative Rx: Low Back Pain
Condition: Acute low back pain
Interventions: Procedure: Acupuncture;
Procedure: Chiropractic;
Procedure: Massage

58 Recruiting

Individualized Chiropractic and Integrative Care for Low Back Pain
Condition: Subacute and chronic low back pain
Interventions: Other: Chiropractic care;
Other: Multidisciplinary, integrative care

68 Recruiting

Dose of Spinal Manipulation for Chronic Low Back Pain
Condition: Low back pain
Interventions: Procedure: Spinal manipulation;
Procedure: Light massage;
Procedure: Pulsed ultrasound

70 Recruiting   **How Does Manual Therapy Improve Low Back Pain for Soldiers?**
Condition: Low back pain
Interventions: Procedure: Soft tissue;
Procedure: Myofascial release;
Procedure: Counterstrain;
Procedure: Muscle energy;
Procedure: Sacroiliac articulation;
Procedure: High-velocity, low amplitude

81 Completed   **Pilot Study to Test the Effectiveness of Combining Conventional and Complementary Medicine to Treat Low Back Pain**
Condition: Low back pain
Interventions: Behavioral: Integrative care for low back pain;
Behavioral: Conventional treatment for low back pain

93 Not yet recruiting   **Chiropractic Management of Chronic Lower Back Pain in Older Adults**
Condition: Chronic lower back pain
Intervention: Procedure: Spinal manipulation

96 Completed   **A Randomized Controlled Trial of Best Approach to Care Compared to Diversified Chiropractic Adjustive Technique**
Conditions: Low back pain; headache; shoulder pain
Intervention: Procedure: spinal manipulation and patient education/nutrition

108 Not yet recruiting   **Education/Exercise and Chiropractic for Chronic Back Pain**
Condition: Low back pain
Interventions: Behavioral: Education and exercise;
Procedure: Chiropractic treatment (plus education and exercise)

123 Recruiting   Chiropractic Prone Distraction for Lower Back Pain
Conditions: Herniated disc; lower back pain; sciatica
Interventions: Procedure: Prone distraction;
Procedure: Side-posture manipulation;
Procedure: Side-posture manipulation and prone distraction;
Procedure: Usual care (control group)

127 Active,   Predicting Patients' Response to Spinal Manipulation
not recruiting   Condition: Low back pain
Intervention: Procedure: Spinal manipulation

Cervical Studies

Thirty-one studies were listed in this category in December 2007. The following have a chiropractic focus:

3 Completed   Manipulation, Exercise, and Self-Care for Neck Pain
Condition: Neck pain
Interventions: Procedure: Chiropractic + Supervised
Rehabilitative Exercise; Procedure: Supervised Rehabilitative Exercise; Behavioral: Self-care education

4 Completed   Randomized Controlled Trial of Chiropractic Manipulation Versus Medical Therapy for Chronic Neck Pain
Condition: Neck pain
Interventions: Procedure: Chiropractic manipulation;
Drug: Acetaminophen

5 Active,   Chiropractic and Exercise for Seniors with
not recruiting   Neck Pain
Condition: Neck pain
Interventions: Procedure: Chiropractic manual treatment
+ home exercise (procedure + behavior);
Procedure: Supervised rehabilitative exercise
+ home exercise;
Behavioral: Home exercise

7 Recruiting **Comparison of the Effectiveness of Mobilization and Manipulation of the Thoracic Spine in Patients with Mechanical Neck Pain**
Condition: Neck pain
Interventions: Procedure: Spine mobilizations;
Procedure: Spine manipulations

10 Active, **Chiropractic Care, Medication, and Self-Care for**
not recruiting **Neck Pain**
Condition: Neck pain
Interventions: Procedure: Chiropractic spinal manipulation;
Drug: Acetaminophen;
Behavioral: Self-care;
Drug: Nonsteroidal anti-inflammatory drugs (NSAIDs);
Drug: Tylenol with codeine

13 Recruiting **Patients with Neck Pain Likely to Benefit from Thoracic Spine Thrust Manipulation**
Condition: Neck pain
Intervention: Other: Thoracic mobilization/manipulation

14 Recruiting **Preventive Care of Chronic Cervical Pain and Disabilities**
Condition: Neck pain
Interventions: Other: Spinal manipulation;
Other: Spinal manipulation + exercises

Headache Studies

Two hundred five studies were listed in this category in December 2007. The following have a chiropractic focus:

45 Completed **Spinal Manipulation for Treatment of Chronic Headaches**
Condition: Headache Disorders
Interventions: Procedure: massage;
Procedure: massage;
Procedure: Spinal manipulation;
Procedure: Spinal manipulation

109 Completed   **A Randomized Controlled Trial of Best Approach to Care Compared to Diversified Chiropractic Adjustive Technique**
Conditions: Low back pain; headache; shoulder pain
Intervention: Procedure: spinal manipulation and
patient education/nutrition[1]

The Bone and Joint Decade 2000–2010 Task Force on Neck Pain and Its Associated Disorders

The president of the Task Force on Neck Pain is Dr. Scott Haldeman, DC, MD, PhD, FCCS(C), FRCP(C), a notable expert on spinal manipulation and safety. The following is taken from the Bone and Joint Decade 2000–2010 Task Force on Neck Pain and Its Associated Disorders Web site:

> *This task force is made up of scientists and clinicians from multiple countries and includes members with diverse training in many of the clinical disciplines that actively treat patients with neck pain. The hope of the Task Force is to help clarify many of the areas of confusion and ignorance and present an up-to-date presentation of our current level of knowledge and understanding of this topic. . . .*
>
> *The task force will address the economic consequences, risk and prevention measures, diagnosis, prognosis, treatment and rehabilitation of neck pain and its associated disorders. The mandate of the task force is to recommend clinical practice guidelines for the management of neck pain and its associated disorders.*"[2]

At the time of publication, the findings were not yet released. It is very likely they will be released soon. As such, it is highly recommended that you search for the status of this study by visiting the Web site of the task force at http://www.nptf.ualberta.ca/.

Aligned Methods (www.alignedmethods.com) will also continue to anticipate the publication of the Task Force findings and findings for many other research projects and to comment on them from a promotional perspective as they are published in the members section.

REFERENCES

1. ClinicalTrials.gov. Home page. Available at http:/www.clinicaltrials.gov. Accessed January 24, 2008.
2. The Bone and Joint Decade 2000–2010 Task Force on Neck Pain and Its Associated Disorders. Available at http://www.nptf.ualberta.ca/

Sample Prescription Pad Information

Acampora Chiropractic Clinic

YOUR APPOINTMENT IS SCHEDULED FOR:

Day: _____   Date: _____   Time: _____

To be completed by the physician's front desk

Patient Name _____

Patient Date of Birth _____

Insurance _____

Is a primary Physician Referral necessary?   ❏ Yes   ❏ No

Referring Physician Name: _____

Referring Physician Phone: _____

To be completed by the referring physician

Clinical Information:

_____

_____

_____

X-Ray or Special Studies: ❏ Yes   ❏ No

If Yes, when were they taken and where can copies be obtained:

_____

Physician Signature _____   Date _____

Patient Information

Your appointment time is noted above. If you are unable to make your scheduled appointment, please contact our office at (888) 555-1212. Please arrive 10 minutes prior to your scheduled appointment to allow time for paperwork. A map of our location, business hours, and contact information are located on the reverse side.

Acampora Chiropractic Clinic

Business Hours: Monday through Fridays 8 A.M. to 6 P.M.
Saturdays by appointment.

555 Lincoln Avenue, Prarieshire, IL 68234
Telephone: (888) 555-1212
Fax: (888) 555-1313
Web site: www.alignedmethods.com

[Insert map or directions to your office. If you are ordering prescription pads for a specific physician, you can place the physician's location on the map as well.]

Note: This prescription pad allows space for the physician's office to schedule the patient's first appointment directly with your office. Requesting that the physician's office make the first appointment for the patient ensures patient compliance.

Sample Summary of Care Letter

To be sent to the referring physician when the patient has completed care.

Date

Referring Physician
Referring Physician Address
Referring Physician City, State, and Zip Code
Regarding: *Patient Name*
DOB: *Patient's Date of Birth*

Dear Dr. *(Referring Physician)*,

Thank you for referring *(Patient's name)* for chiropractic care to my offices for *(list general condition, such as lower back pain)*. Enclosed is an updated summary of his/her treatment outcome.

History

(Mr./Ms. Patient's name) presented for care on *(date)* for *(general condition, list any radiculopathy)* of *(duration of condition such as "6 weeks duration")*. *(Mr./Ms. Patient's name)* describes the pain as *(describe the patient's pain such as intermittent, constant, moderate, sharp, achey, and so on)*. *(Mr./Ms. Patient's name)* indicates that the pain is made better/worse *(list any situations that exacerbate or bring the patient relief)* and *(he/she)* has limitations in *(his/her)* activities of daily living such as *(describe what the patient doesn't do or avoids because of the condition)*.

Objective findings include *(list any scoring tests such as a Visual Analog score, Oswestry Disability score, Roland-Morris score, and so on.*

Make sure to qualify the score such as a Visual Analog score of 6 out of 10 or an Oswestry Disability score consistent with moderate disability).

(Mr./Ms. Patient's name) had *(list objective findings. It is not necessary to list all orthopedic tests and specific range of motion findings unless you determine that the doctor prefers to have them listed. The following will do for a summary report:* "*Upon examination Mrs. Acampora had bilateral paraspinal spasm and tenderness more notable on the right, difficulty rising from a seated position and painful endrange motion with right lumbar rotation. Some mild swelling was noted to the right of her lumbosacral junction. Kemp's testing was positive on the right for moderate pain.*").

Treatment Summary

(Patient Name) received *(number of sessions)* over *(number of weeks),* which included manipulation to the *(indicate the area of the spine; if you treat a lumbar condition with full spine manipulation, you should educate the doctor in advance as to the reason why; otherwise, the doctor may question why you manipulated the cervical region for a lumbar patient),* regional soft tissue work, ergonomic and exercise instruction for active home care. Ice was initially indicated due to the presence of swelling *(or any physical therapy modality and the physiological finding prompting you to provide it).* (Mr./Ms. Patient name) was encouraged to remain active and to assist in *(his/her)* own care through stretching and specific exercises provided in the initial treatment consultation.

Discharge Findings

On *(date, which should match the date of this type of letter)* *(Patient Name)* was discharged from care with the following subjective and objective findings: *(list any remaining objective findings; minor findings such as a small localized area of tenderness are not necessary as long as it is listed in your treatment notes).* Upon discharge *(Mr./Ms. Patient name)* reported that there were no limitations on *(his/her)* activities of daily living *(or list any remaining limitations if this patient is permanent and stationary).* (Mr./Ms. Patient name) had a *(provide updated outcome measurement assessment test values such as a Visual Analog Scale of 0 on a pain scale of 10 or an Oswestry Disability score consistent with minimal disability).*

Impressions

(Patient Name) has achieved full recovery with no residuals *(or list permanent and stationary and any residual findings or list remaining residuals).*

Recommendations

(Mr./Mrs. Patient Name) was discharged and encouraged to continue exercises to maintain strength and prevent reoccurrence *(or, patient was discharged and advised to return for care as needed for flare-ups over and above his/her permanent and stationary levels or list the need and plan for continued care).*

Thank you again for referring this patient to my office. Should you have any questions, please feel free to contact me at *(your telephone number).*

Sincerely,

Chiropractor Name, DC

- For those chiropractors with electronic medical records, these reports are extremely quick and easy to generate. If you share the same software as the referring physician, it is even easier because the reports can be transmitted electronically.
- Remember from Chapter 7 that physicians don't want every detail, just an overview. Keep the report concise and to the point and avoid words such as *subluxation, trigger points,* and so on.

Variations on the Letter

To keep overall length short, the history may be omitted and a one-line sentence describing the pain may be substituted such as the following: *"Patient presents with nontraumatic, insidious moderate right lower back pain of 6 weeks, which has not improved with time."*

Index

Note: Italic indicators refer to figures.

N

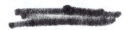

CPSIA information can be obtained
at www.ICGtesting.com
Printed in the USA
FFHW011657150919
54914409-60640FF